Careers
in
Veterinary Surgery

Careers
in
Veterinary Surgery

Vivien Donald

**Kogan
Page**

Acknowledgements

The author would like to thank the many busy veterinary surgeons who gave up their time to describe their many different types of work, in the UK and overseas.

First published 1985 by Kogan Page Limited
120 Pentonville Road, London N1 9JN

British Library Cataloguing in Publication Data
Donald, Vivien
    Careers in veterinary surgery.
    1. Veterinary medicine — Vocational guidance —
    Great Britain
    I. Title
    636.089'023'41   SF756.28

    ISBN 0 85038 957 7

Printed and bound in Great Britain by
The Camelot Press Ltd, Southampton

Contents

Part 2

Introduction

Although about half the qualified veterinary surgeons in the UK spend their days coping with pets who cannot describe their symptoms, and who may bite if asked, or delving into the back ends of cows on behalf of profit-conscious farmers, there are other types of work open to a qualified veterinary surgeon that do not involve the actual treatment of animals. A great deal of importance is attached nowadays to the prevention and control of animal diseases, as opposed to their diagnosis and treatment, not only for domestic animals but mainly within the agriculture industry, and this involves research, and also Ministry and local authority work.

The vet who is working within a private practice will often combine both agricultural and domestic animal care, in what is known as a 'mixed' practice. A 'small animal' practice deals with domestic pets, probably in a large town. The pets to be cared for may be as small as goldfish, gerbils and budgerigars, and may include reptiles such as snakes and terrapins, as well as cats and dogs. The vet will make house calls during his or her daily routine, but many of the animals will be seen in the practice's surgery. The vet becomes closely involved with the pet owners themselves, often young children or the very elderly, who are strongly attached to their companions, and a sympathetic skill in dealing with people can be as important to a vet as a love of animals and dedication to their welfare.

The agricultural or large animal practice takes the vet round the farms and fields. There is a great deal of travelling around the countryside, pregnancy testing and blood testing cows and pigs. Handling large, heavy animals can be demanding physically and all veterinary surgeons must experience it at some time, as part of their training. However, it is certainly not too tough for women to manage, and about one-third of the students on veterinary degree courses are women (1983-4 figures).

Competition for places on these courses is strong. In the UK there are six universities offering veterinary training, and the course lasts five or six years, depending on the university. Entry qualifications are high (see Chapter 7) and competition is fierce, so some experience of working with animals during school holidays, either on a farm, in kennels or in a vet's surgery, will help applicants. It will also give them the chance to decide whether a career as a vet really suits them — for instance, it may happen that an allergy to animals becomes apparent during work of this kind.

Once training is completed, the graduate becomes a member of the Royal College of Veterinary Surgeons, and is then free to practise. Most will enter a practice as a veterinary assistant, and will move around between practices to gain experience; eventually they will become a partner in a practice, buy a practice, or begin a new one. Usually there are three or four vets and one or two partners within one practice, so that there can be one or more 'on call' 24 hours a day, every day, and partners may specialise in, for instance, horses, livestock or small animals.

Other branches of the veterinary profession include the State Veterinary Service, either a part of the Ministry of Agriculture, Fisheries and Food (MAFF) in England and Wales, or the Department of Agriculture and Fisheries in Scotland (DAFS), and the environmental health departments of local authorities. The work is concerned with detecting and controlling diseases such as brucellosis and foot and mouth, and with meat hygiene, public health and the improvement of animal welfare on farms, in kennels, pet shops, stables and zoos.

Research into animal diseases is carried out in the MAFF and DAFS laboratories, in the university veterinary schools and in private laboratories, often owned by large pharmaceutical companies. There are also several postgraduate courses available in the universities, and these can lead eventually to teaching posts. Qualified veterinary surgeons can also find posts with the Royal Army Veterinary Corps, in developing countries overseas, and in industry and commerce.

Part 1

Chapter 1
Practice Work

The lad who joined the course in veterinary medicine at the University of Edinburgh a few years ago purely on the strength of having read some James Herriot books will have realised long before the end of his five-year course (if he completed it) that his idea of a veterinary surgeon's life was very out of date.

The kind of large animal practice that Herriot was mainly engaged in is shrinking nowadays, and although it still seems to remain as an image of the ideal way of life in the minds of many veterinary surgeons, especially in the summertime when the weather is sunny, they acknowledge that it is no longer economically viable either for the farmers or for the veterinary surgeons. However, if large animal or agricultural practice, as it is sometimes called, is on the decline, small animal practice and work to do with horses is increasing, although the population of companion animals is holding steady. Horses and ponies are companion animals too, and are part of today's rapid growth industry of leisure pursuits. The result is that studs, hunters and family ponies all contribute to the veterinary surgeon's work.

Most practices combine all these types of work, and are known as mixed or general practices, although each of the partners may specialise in one particular aspect such as horses or agricultural work. There are also, however, a large number of practices dealing exclusively with small animals, particularly in towns, and this type is generally thought of as being the most remunerative.

When they leave veterinary college, most graduates

work for two or three years as assistants in at least one, more often two or three, different practices to gain experience and make up their minds about where they want to spend the rest of their working lives. The time spent is useful, even if they then decide to leave practice work and go into research, back into the academic life as teachers, work for a commercial pharmaceutical company producing veterinary products, or work abroad. In fact, just under half of the 12,000 veterinary surgeons on the Royal College's register are working in practice.

Personal Qualities

An understanding and feeling for animals are important for practice work, of course, but being able to deal sympathetically with the general public — and farmers — is invaluable too. Very often it is the owner of a sick pet who is more concerned and upset than the animal itself; and indeed, very often a pet's problem can be bound up with the character of the owner. It is naturally distressing if a companion animal has to be put down when it is incurably ill and in pain, and the veterinary surgeons find that they must necessarily be conscious of and understand their clients' emotions. On the other side of the coin, there is inevitably the problem of dealing diplomatically with difficult clients, and coping with those who refuse to pay their bills.

Physical stamina is also necessary because practice work can involve being on duty for perhaps 36 hours together and very often this can include calls in the middle of the night. It requires a great deal of tact to deal cheerfully with a client whose pet has been looking off-colour all day, but who has left it until late evening to call the vet. Other calls may involve 'fire brigade' emergencies on farms that can mean a long tramp over the fields in the dark, or an examination at the side of the road by the light of a car's headlights on a traffic accident casualty.

Unlike veterinary surgeons who are employed by the Ministry of Agriculture, research institutes, universities or pharmaceutical companies, those who decide on a partnership in practice will be running their own business, and so another requirement is the ability to deal with paperwork and accounts.

How a Practice is Run

There are a few practices run by a single veterinary surgeon, and at the other extreme there is one 17-person practice, but most are run by three or four veterinary surgeons. A practice with several vets means there are fewer weekends and evenings on duty, and more chance to work for periods that are nearer to normal office hours. Normally a partner works about one weekend in three.

In any practice there will be 'lay' workers as well as the veterinary surgeons and these may be animal nursing auxiliaries (who may be fully qualified registered animal nursing auxiliaries) or trainees, plus receptionists and cleaners. The receptionists often work on a rota system, deal with all the telephone calls and appointments and also look after the book-keeping. A large practice may need the services of a full-time business administrator to take the administrative problems off the veterinary surgeons' hands.

Some practices may have three surgeries a day with one of the partners in charge while the others go out making calls. The surgeries may be from 9.00 to 10.00 am, 2.00 to 3.00 pm and an evening surgery from 6.00 to 7.00 pm. More practices, however, have all day surgeries. There are morning and perhaps afternoon surgeries on Saturdays and Sundays as well. Operations may be carried out on two or three days a week, for non-emergency operations such as spaying, castrating and the removal of tumours.

The veterinary surgeons who are out on calls follow an appointments schedule drawn up by the receptionists on the basis of requests made to the surgery the day before or early in the morning. Most vets nowadays have a bleeper or radio telephone system so that they can be contacted on their round and told of any new calls.

The premises may be a part of a partner's home, or have a flat attached for the veterinary surgeon on duty to use overnight or at weekends if animals are hospitalised and need to remain overnight. The surgery will consist of waiting room, consulting room or rooms, office, kennels and cages, and dispensary. Other facilities include operating theatre and X-ray machines, and larger practices may also have a separate laboratory and loose boxes, if there is a great deal of equine work.

Large Animal Practice

Even a practice that deals mainly with large animals will have a few small animals as well. Usually there will be one or more partners within a practice dealing almost exclusively with the large animal work, while his or her colleagues handle the other areas. 'Large animal' is generally taken to mean 'agricultural' or farm animal, and is therefore concerned basically with food production as well as animal welfare. Although there is generally less large animal work now, practices in the traditional dairying areas such as Somerset and Cheshire are still busy and profitable.

Economics plays a large part in the agricultural industry with the result that the farmer has to decide whether or not it is financially worthwhile to treat an animal. If it is going to cost £15 or £20 to treat a calf that is only worth £25, then he or she will either get rid of the calf, or let it take pot luck. If the calf is worth £100, however, it is worth spending £20 on it. Although a cat owner whose pet has broken its leg in a particularly complicated way in a car accident may spend a great deal of money to have the leg put back together again, the calf that breaks its leg ceases to be an economic unit.

Agricultural work is more concerned with preventive medicine, and with disease prevention methods. Herds and flocks undertake regular programmes of vaccination, testing, dipping and drenching so that diseases can be avoided as far as possible. Much of this work is controlled by the Ministry of Agriculture, Fisheries and Food's State Veterinary Service (see Chapter 2), but a great deal of the routine work of tuberculin and brucellosis testing is undertaken by veterinary surgeons in practice who have contracts with the Ministry.

Since farmers have of necessity become more economy-minded, and have also taken to using the hypodermic and so been able to treat and follow-up this treatment themselves, the number of visits made to farms each day has gone down. Veterinary surgeons find they are dealing with a larger number of farm animals and advising on a herd or flock basis and less on a single animal basis. They may be called in by the farmer who is worried about a lack of fertility or performance, but there are no specific symptoms, so it means taking a lot of samples, sending them off to the laboratory, and then collating the results when they arrive. Then the veterinary surgeon and client decide together on a plan of action.

Ministry programmes can also be time-consuming: TB testing means visiting to inject the herd and then visiting again to read the tests. Certain times of the year may be more busy than others. Autumn and spring are busy times with sheep; in the autumn the work includes giving advice to the farmers on their dipping, worming, drenching and feeding programmes for the ewes before lambing time. Lambing time is also busy, although very often ewes needing Caesarians will be taken to the surgery in the back of the farmer's truck. Unfortunately, too, spring and summer involve recovering or killing ewes and lambs that have been worried by dogs, or giving them antibiotic injections.

Dairy herds are also visited on a routine basis if the farmer wishes it; usually weekly or fortnightly to keep an eye on the breeding fertility of the herd, to keep mastitis down and to be aware of changes in environment, weather or feed (especially in winter), to keep an eye on health and performance, and to give advice.

Pigs are normally visited regularly too, maybe 25 times a year, to assess the herd performance, the impact of disease on herd performance, to note any deviations in target performance and to prevent the effects of lost production from disease. Some of this work is now done on an annual contract basis, some in conjunction with pharmaceutical companies in schemes to provide drugs to the farmers with the backing of veterinary advice, if the vet believes it necessary. Veterinary surgeons involved in large animal practice welcome any opportunities they have to visit the farms regularly in an advisory role, rather than on 'fire brigade' visits.

In fact, there are not many emergency visits of the 'drop everything and run' type. Other emergencies may involve a twisted gut, a prolapsed uterus, a broken leg, acute poisoning, magnesium deficiency or difficulty in calving, which would call for operations on the farm. Other more routine visits to farms would be for debudding of horns, castrating and pregnancy testing.

Small Animal Practice

Practices dealing with companion animals alone are normally in the larger towns, or villages with a high proportion of pet-owning families, and they can be very profitable for the veterinary surgeon. Large villages of 10,000 in some areas, however, easily support a small animal practice. Whereas the farmers must consider economic factors in treating their animals, a pet owner who has acquired a kitten, perhaps for nothing, may spend enormous amounts on it for sentimental reasons. Because these owners on the whole are prepared to spend money on their animals, the opportunities for sophisticated techniques are sometimes greater. The veterinary surgeon can develop skills in specialised areas of surgery because there are fewer financial restraints.

It can be more pleasant and satisfying to spend a day in the surgery working with animals all the time, but the outlay on premises and the necessity of having larger numbers of lay staff and greater overheads increase costs. More small animal practices are operated single-handedly, or are a two-person partnership, than in the mixed practices.

The small animal practice is a relatively new phenom-enon but has made great strides in recent years, taking the level of treatment virtually to the human level. Over 70 have met requirements laid down by the Royal College and are able to call their surgeries 'veterinary hospitals'. With the increasingly sophisticated equipment, small animal veterinary surgeons are able to treat animals that previously they would have had to put down, or send to one of the veterinary schools for further diagnosis.

In small animal practice, less of the day is spent in making house calls than in large or mixed practices, and more in consultations at the surgery and in doing oper-ations. House calls are discouraged because there are none of the diagnostic facilities and trained assistants available, as there are at the surgery, and because the owners are often unwilling to pay for the extra time involved in a house call.

The consultations with the owner are the times when veterinary practice becomes a job that is virtually more to do with people than with animals. It is important to deal with the pet owners, who may be children, with patience and understanding and get them to describe the animal's symptoms clearly. Like farmers, the pet owners are usually loyal clients, and so it becomes possible to get to know individual animals and learn about their home environ-ment, which makes diagnosis easier, and it is satisfying to be able to follow the animal's progress and recovery. The examination of the animal can be a tricky time, especially when one is dealing with an uncertain-tempered dog who does not take kindly to being touched in a painful spot.

It is also important to be able to explain the treatment to owners, and get them to co-operate. Very often these days the animals are overweight, and it is not always easy to stop fond owners from feeding up their sick pets with too many doggy chocs and biscuits. Part of a veterinary surgeon's job in this area is putting over the idea of responsible pet ownership to the clients, and getting them to stick to a sensible routine of diet, exercise and vaccinations.

Practices with hospitals attached can admit animals to

the hospital for more extensive diagnosis or for surgery. The surgery may be the routine neutering of cats and dogs, but very often it can be more interesting and satisfying: correcting hip dysplasia in a pedigree dog, removing dangerous tumours, even replacing an arthritic hip joint. Operations and hospitalisation can be expensive for the owner, but it is very fulfilling when an operation means that a much-loved family pet is restored to good health and a longer life.

Animal patients that cannot be helped by the practice facilities can be referred to another veterinary practice or to the specialists at one of the veterinary schools. Skin cases, for instance, can be intractable problems, very often with no cure. The clients often want a second opinion, and rather than have them visit another vet stealthily, their own vet will suggest that the animal should be examined by a specialist in dermatology. It gives the client peace of mind, even though the answer will still be that nothing more can be done. Skin problems are not always incurable. Often a few questions from the vet reveal that it has moved to a new environment — maybe a town dog is on holiday by the sea and is just not used to sand and sea salt. (Veterinary practices in holiday areas can be particularly busy during the summer season, when there is a lull in agricultural work.)

The veterinary school specialists can cope with more dramatic cases than skin disorders, and the cost to the client is not inordinately high because the costs are heavily subsidised. A consultation costs about £10 (plus travelling costs for the patient and owner, of course). Even an open-heart operation with three experienced cardiologists involved may cost only about £100. An example of this kind of operation involved an elderly single lady and a puppy who was perfectly healthy apart from a congenital heart defect; to the veterinary surgeon it was obvious that the owner had become emotionally dependent on her companion and so the case seemed worth proceeding with, and was highly successful.

In a progressive small animal practice the partners

continue to improve their skills and facilities and a considerable proportion of the profits must be ploughed back into the practice to buy the necessary X-ray equipment, ultrasonic dental scalers, anaesthetic machines, etc. The partners will also regularly attend courses to keep up with the latest techniques.

In general practice a veterinary surgeon may average between six and ten consultations per day, plus perhaps five visits and two operations, and could be either working non-stop for 24 hours or drinking coffee and sitting about during slack times. In a small animal practice he or she would average between 25 and 30 consultations per day, and perhaps five operations. The work is more structured but there are more people to deal with and it involves more evening work.

Dogs and cats make up the majority of small animal patients, but there is a much greater variety of other species than are seen in farm animal work. Budgerigars and other cage birds are popular, too, and the veterinary surgeon finds him or herself diagnosing and treating not only the guinea pigs, rabbits, mice and gerbils that children have as pets, but also monkeys, terrapins, snakes and tropical fish. In this kind of practice there is the chance to specialise in a particular interest almost as a hobby, but use the knowledge to help the practice. It means, too, that there is a great variety in the work each day, with calls from, for instance, the owner of a Great Dane that has swallowed a child's lollipop, stick and all, or the treating of a jackdaw with a split beak. It can even mean, as in one case, treating a seal, that had been living happily for months in a local river until it became ill and was brought to the surgery by the local ambulancemen in their ambulance (the stretcher was just the right size); it was diagnosed as having pneumonia, pumped full of penicillin and was soon able to go back to the sea.

Equine Practice

A smattering of geological knowledge helps in pinpointing

the types of equine work around the country, as the top stud farms are concentrated in chalk and limestone areas, including where the North and South Downs meet, Salisbury Plain, Lambourne, Newbury, Newmarket and right up to Yorkshire, where the limestone pavement ends. This is because the soil is well-drained and produces good going for racing. In these areas there are veterinary surgeons who deal only with the very expensive horses.

In the South East and Home Counties, there is a concentration of 'pleasure' horses used for eventing and hunting, and also children's ponies.

There are very few trainers who employ full-time vets, although all the best trainers will have one or two vets in their yard every day. They visit routinely to monitor the horses' general health, take blood samples to check for virus disorders and make any other tests necessary as a form of preventive medicine; they also attend the yard as and when required.

The busy time on stud farms is in January, when the mares are foaling. Work for a stud will involve all the more usual horse illnesses, as well as diseases in the foals and young horses, disease especially relating to brood mares, investigating abortion, difficulties in maintaining pregnancy, assistance at foaling time, routine pregnancy testing (important from an economic point of view as the stallion's stud fees are paid in two instalments, the last on a second pregnancy test in October), tetanus vaccination, prevention of worm infestation and taking bacteriological swabs before a mare goes away to be covered to prevent her carrying disease to the stud.

Everyday pleasure horses are not such a problem for their owners because they are not so highly bred. With children's ponies, veterinary surgeons are most busy coping with laminitis and sweet itch, but ponies in general are tougher and require less attention unless there are accidents with wire on the hunting field requiring stitch-ups, or lameness.

One of the biggest growth areas in recent years has been eventing, which means that veterinary surgeons must attend the events and trials, and many Saturdays and Sundays are spent standing around, often unpaid, at horse trials in case a horse is injured. Polo requires the same sort of weekend duty.

Legislation is being discussed that could outlaw fox-hunting in the future, but drag racing will still take place — and in fact can be worse for the horses as it involves a lot of flat-out racing and no periods standing around doing nothing, so the veterinary surgeon will continue to find himself working with hunters.

Wholly equine practices may have their own hospitals attached but, because the capital required is very large for major operating facilities, the difficult types of surgery are usually better carried out at the teaching hospitals which already have the best conditions and facilities for large animals. Hospitals attached to equine practices are generally for recovery, and the owners normally like to care for their horses at home as soon as they can walk.

As the horse population of the country has been estimated at around half a million there is a great deal of work in this area for veterinary surgeons, and very often one partner in a mixed or agricultural practice will specialise in horse and pony work.

Specialisation

In a mixed practice partners tend to concentrate on one type of work, although they can all cover for each other if necessary. So within a practice one partner will deal mainly with the farm livestock, another perhaps with horses, and so on. This gives them the chance to keep up to date with the latest knowledge about their subject, and attend courses and seminars that are of particular interest to them. With the advance of knowledge in all fields, it is virtually impossible for the general practitioner to keep up to date in all areas.

Specialisation depends on what goes on within the practice's catchment area. If there is a mink farm, or fish farms, the veterinary surgeons extend their knowledge of mink and fish by reading up on the subject as well as attending any courses available. If there is a large poultry farm in the area, it obviously makes sense to specialise in poultry, and one of the partners may be dealing with poultry work virtually full time. The same may apply to pig work.

Some practices may act as consultants to greyhound stadiums. Veterinary surgeons must attend all greyhound race meetings and trials meetings held under the rules of the National Greyhound Racing Club, just as they must also attend horse racing meetings. They look after the dogs' welfare and make sure that if any are not fit to race, they are withdrawn. All dogs are pre-race examined twice, once at kennelling and once about 15 minutes before the 'off' to check that they are not lame or obviously ill, since it would not be fair either to the dog or the people attending the meeting to run a dog in poor condition. The veterinary surgeons stay in the kennel area or within the stadium, watch the races and check the dogs again as they come off the track. There are also a few vets employed full time by the Greyhound Racing Association.

Other establishments within a practice's area can bring the veterinary surgeon in touch with more exotic animals. For instance, there may be a zoo or safari park that employs the local veterinary surgeons on a consultancy basis, rather than having one working for them full time. Travelling circuses and circus animals wintered out on local farms provide variety, too. A bad-tempered llama whose toe-nails need to be cut, a constipated elephant, or a lion with toothache cannot fail to provide a touch of variety in a vet's life. In cases such as this, he or she can phone other veterinarians used to zoo animals for advice, if necessary, on how much anaesthetic to use, or whatever.

Specialisation in all areas of veterinary medicine is on the increase, and for the veterinary surgeon in practice it not only means becoming more involved with one or two particular species, but also learning about advances in technology and expertise.

There are various courses where veterinary surgeons can

gain a diploma, but this does mean extra work and extra-mural study. There are full-time one-year courses at certain universities, short courses, and a series of lectures at the British Veterinary Association's annual congress that acts as an updating programme. In general practice, courses can be selected that cover a special interest within the practice, and subjects include radiology, anaesthesia, oph-thalmology, cattle infertility, animal nutrition, etc. The pharmaceutical companies also run courses on subjects connected with their products.

Working for the Ministry of Agriculture or Local Authority

Many veterinary surgeons working in general practice are employed on a contract basis by the Ministry of Agriculture, Fisheries and Food (MAFF) or the local authority. Those employed by MAFF are known as Local Veterinary Inspec-tors (LVIs) and carry out most of the routine tuberculin testing and brucellosis sampling required by the Ministry, and would also help in eradicating local outbreaks of serious diseases such as foot and mouth or swine vesicular disease.

Very few local authorities employ full-time vets, but they must employ them on a contractual basis to carry out certain legal requirements. Meat hygiene is one important area of responsibility. The local authorities are responsible for meat inspection by law, and where there is red meat for export there must be veterinary supervision for meat inspection and general hygiene. The local authorities have to provide that service and must appoint a veterinary surgeon at abattoirs, who has overall responsibility for administration and welfare. Some of the work is on behalf of MAFF, such as residue testing, and certification. This type of work, of course, depends on whether there is an abattoir in the vicinity — not all towns will have one. The workload depends on the throughput of the abattoir, but the vet must be there at all times when it is dealing with red meat for export.

The local authority appoints either a practice or an individual veterinary surgeon to do the work for them, and the vet or practice must be designated as fit to do it by MAFF. The hourly rate works out at around £12.50, which is not considered a good income for a veterinary surgeon. A contract with an abattoir can work out at around £25,000 to £30,000 annually, but as this would include the time of at least two veterinary surgeons, including holidays and extras, it is not highly remunerative. Hours are variable: in one practice there may be someone working full time, 40 or 50 hours per week; at others it may be as low as five hours per week — it depends on the local markets.

Two other areas of work for local authorities that are undertaken by veterinary surgeons in general practice are the inspection of meat products for export, and poultry. There must be an official veterinary surgeon for any poultry-processing plant, but in this case full-time attendance is not necessary.

In addition, the local authority is responsible for the licensing of dog breeders, riding establishments, boarding kennels, pet shops, zoos and anyone keeping dangerous wild animals, and employ local veterinary surgeons to make inspections on their behalf.

Other Types of Supplementary Work

Often veterinary surgeons in practice are asked by pharmaceutical companies to take part in field trials of new products, or to advise farmers on the use of their new products. They also treat animals on a contract basis for the welfare societies (see Chapter 5). Teaching is also possible, as general practitioners may be asked to lecture to students by the Agricultural Training Board or at agricultural colleges.

Students

As students must spend a period of six months with a

veterinary practice towards the end of their course, many practices have a student working with them and learning from them at some time during the vacations. They travel around on calls, as well as gaining practical experience at the surgery premises.

Assistants

As soon as they leave veterinary school, most new graduates work as assistants in a practice. Although new graduates do not have a wealth of experience, they frequently have certain skills and expertise — for instance in laboratory diagnosis techniques — which a practice with a sophisticated laboratory would like to acquire. The starting salary is from about £7,000, but this varies according to the type of practice (small animal practices may pay more). Practices looking for assistants advertise in the *Veterinary Record*, the magazine published by the British Veterinary Association. Normally a flat or small house and car are provided. Once the graduate has some practice experience, he or she can move on to other practices, and the salary may be £10,000 to £12,000 a year.

Very occasionally partnerships ask for a married — or cohabiting — assistant, because they want someone who will be able to answer the telephone during the evenings and weekends when the assistant is on duty. They normally offer four weeks' holiday and the hours would include at least one night a week on call, and one Sunday in four. Sometimes the advertisement will be for an assistant 'with a view to partnership', and working as an assistant can be a good way into eventual partnership. But practice work does involve long hours, on an average 80 hours per week, because there must always be someone available 24 hours a day, seven days a week, and graduates may decide at this stage to go into research or apply to work for MAFF or one of the pharmaceutical companies where the hours are not so long.

Working as an assistant gives you a chance to understand the business side of running a practice, and it helps a great deal if the partners give assistants an idea of such things as cash flow, overheads and how much things cost and give them the chance to do their own pricing so that they can understand the pricing structure of the business. If the principal partner always handles the business side of the practice himself or herself, the assistant can leave without ever having learned about it. It also helps an assistant to understand that some people are bad debts, and to become a judge of character, if possible, and recognise the people who are likely to be bad payers, or have been in the past.

The BVA has drawn up a suggested form of agreement between principals and assistants to help avoid problems connected with such things as insurance, pensions, use of the car, holidays, sickness, hours of duty and length of service. The BVA strongly recommends that a contract between a principal and assistant should be drawn up and signed, regulating the terms of the employment, to avoid any confusions arising.

Under the terms of the Contracts of Employment Act 1972, it is the responsibility of the employer to provide the employee with a written statement of the main terms and conditions of employment within 13 weeks of the employee starting work.

The principal and assistant must also come to an agreement about what happens after the term of service is finished; usually a 'binding out' clause is included in the agreement to prevent the assistant setting up his or her own practice in the same area, and this involves deciding on how large an area should be considered, and for how many years. If the assistant intended to start a totally different type of practice, that would not conflict with his principal's, these strictures may not apply.

The leaflet published by the BVA, 'Model agreements between principals and assistants', gives further advice (price £1.00).

Salaried Partners

A practice sometimes takes on an assistant and calls him a

'salaried partner', mainly to make him or her seem more acceptable to the clients. The assistant normally gets an additional bonus on top of his agreed salary. However, the BVA warns that the existence of the salaried partner's name on the notepaper means he could be liable for the partnership's debts, even though he is not in fact a full partner, and they strongly advise against becoming a salaried partner.

Going into Partnership

The established way of going into practice is that one leaves the one, two or three practices where one has worked as an assistant, and then joins an establishment as an assistant with a view to partnership. An established practice will have a well-worn way of retiring partners who have reached retiring age, and taking on new ones, and so the practice continues. This is a less expensive way of becoming a partner than buying a practice and premises outright, but there is still a fairly large outlay involved, as the new partner will have to buy his or her way in, and will need some sort of loan for financing the enterprise. The new partner buys assets such as fixtures and fittings, good debts, car, equipment, drugs and premises, including houses. Normally a valuation of the practice property is carried out when a new partner is taken into a practice. Obviously the amount the new partner will have to pay varies a great deal between practices, but the sum could be around £18,000. In the past new partners also had to buy goodwill, which might have taken such a sum up to around £60,000. If the new partner has been working as an assistant in the practice, and so helped to build up goodwill, there is usually a reduction in his or her share.

Goodwill may consist simply of the right to circulate the practice's clients informing them that it has changed ownership, or it may represent the value of taking over, or becoming a partner in and so sharing the profits of an efficient, progressive and profitable practice. Though some practices have abandoned it altogether, most new partners still have to buy goodwill, but instead of buying it outright there is a trend towards providing the outgoing partner or his or her family with an annuity, or pension, which is based on what the goodwill was worth. For instance, a retiring partner's share of the practice could be £31,000. His or her share of the assets (fixtures and fittings, and so on) might be valued at £8,000, so the goodwill is reckoned to be worth £23,000. The pension, therefore, is based on an investment of £23,000, providing an income of £2,300 annually, paid by the practice and charged against tax. (New partners should also make arrangements for their own pensions, to guard against inflation.) The initial cost of buying goodwill can also be reduced if the new partner accepts reduced earnings for a few years before coming into full partnership.

Partners have a two-year period after a change in partnership during which they can decide whether they wish the partnership to continue. Very often partners find that they simply cannot work amicably together, although this problem can sometimes be overcome if the partners specialise in different areas of work, or even work from different branch surgeries.

Of course, before anyone signs any agreement on a partnership, the legal and financial aspects must be discussed with his or her own solicitor and accountant. First the practice's solicitor and accountant are usually consulted, and before any final agreement is reached, there will be a draft agreement submitted to the new partner by the existing partnership.

After 10 to 15 years in a successful practice, a partner could be grossing around £35,000 — way over the equivalent in the industrial world.

The BVA leaflet, 'Guide to partnerships in veterinary practice', goes into the implications of partnerships in great detail, and gives a helpful guide to the value of goodwill (price £1.00).

Practices for Sale

Advertisements for practices for sale can be found in the

Veterinary Record. Buying outright is a more expensive way of taking over a practice, and means you must be able to run a business successfully, cope with financial aspects, employ staff and deal with the paperwork. It is also important to be forward-looking, keeping up with developments and new technology and investing, if necessary, in expensive new equipment.

As small animal practice is the most profitable normally, it may be better to consider this kind of practice, taking into account where it is situated, and whether there seem to be plenty of possible clients in the area. Although large animal practice is shrinking, a new housing estate in the area could mean that it would be possible to change from agricultural to companion animal work.

It is also sensible to look at the geographical area, and decide whether travelling time could affect profitability.

Prices for practices vary enormously. For example, a price was advertised for a practice for two partners or principal plus assistant in the Midlands of around £64,000, including freehold surgery premises, with flat, goodwill, instruments and equipment. A similar practice in Scotland, with a turnover of around £55,000, was advertised at around £61,000. If a large stock of drugs is included in the assets, the asking price might be higher.

Women in Practice

There are very few farmers today who are prejudiced against women veterinary surgeons, and women who do go into large animal practice are usually considered to be very good indeed because of their dedication. Handling farm animals is normally done by the stockman when the vet calls anyway. Sometimes the hours of small animal practice suit a woman who has family responsibilities, and a practice which has several partners would be more suitable than a small practice, where there may be more difficulty in getting someone to cover for absence.

Married women often find that the office hours of MAFF veterinary investigation centres are more suitable;

or in pharmaceutical companies, especially as there are better prospects now of promotion for women within large companies.

Research in Practice

Although there are no opportunities for pure research in practice, there are some veterinary surgeons who are well known for work they have done; one veterinary surgeon has done a great deal of important work in equine fertility, as well as running a busy equine practice. One may also be at the forefront of new diseases that appear, and know more about them from clinical observation than veterinary surgeons in the laboratories. A general practitioner who is very interested in a subject can read up on it, discuss it with colleagues and do some useful and practical research of his or her own.

Case Studies

Nick is a new partner in a mixed practice.

I went to Cambridge and part-way through my course did a degree in the economics of agriculture. I also did three months' research in economics and epidemiology at Reading University. I tried to get a broad experience during the vacations. I had a scholarship to study dairying in Israel, then did an expedition to the little islands in the Arctic to study avian influenza in the wild bird population there. I went to Zambia under the auspices of the World Health Organisation to work with the Save the Rhino Trust, worked on a pig farm in Denmark, and also at a stud in Newmarket. After Cambridge I did a short course on fish pathology at Stirling, which I use quite a lot now because there are four fish farms in the area. I then worked for a mixed practice for five years, which included fish farm work, and was also good on horses, with operating surgeries, and so on. Then I came to my present practice where about 80 per cent of my work is with horses.

I start work at 8.30 am. Some people telephone me at home before I start work, at about 8.00 am, so parts of the day and certain visits are already organised. A typical day would include visiting sick horses, worming some, stitching up horses with bad cuts (during the hunting season), going to see a horse that is hopping lame and admitting it for X-ray at the surgery, giving tetanus jabs, rasping teeth and seeing horses with respiratory problems. As well as looking at horses I'll also be asked to look at small animals as well — maybe a chicken and a rabbit and some pheasants that need treating — plus doing the odd small animal house call if there is one that needs a visit and there is no one else in the practice available to make it. I'll get home at around 9.00 pm.

Practice work is very enjoyable, but the hours are long. It offers a great challenge and you can make use of an enormous amount of your training, but it's a hard life — piece work, really. You only get paid for what you do, and you've got to turn out day and night in order to provide the service. It's quite hard physically and with the hours spent on call it adds up to about 80 hours a week.

Tim is principal partner in a mixed practice.

If you want a practice to be successful it is important to belong to the community — belong to the NFU, do something with the Young Farmers, talk to the WI, lecture for the Agricultural Training Board, and so on. If you do nothing in that line, people don't know you exist. It also helps to have new and energetic blood in the practice and to cover specialist areas.

I thought of going into the Royal Army Veterinary Corps, but having spent six weeks with them over a couple of years I decided there just wasn't enough veterinary work, and you would come out having lost ground however long you were in — even two years — as far as knowledge of practice work was concerned. I would love to swap a year with a Canadian veterinary surgeon, but out there the small animal practices are mainly in the populated areas and large animal practices are up in the north, so there are very few who are doing truly mixed practice, as I am.

Michael is in a small animal practice.

I came here from a mixed practice and, although I was only four years out of College, I really had to brush up my medicine to get used to the very sophisticated techniques here. I want to specialise and will work for a diploma in dermatology. I think a lot of the public would be surprised how little like James Herriot practice work is; you've got to be up to date with your techniques and there's a lot of expense and machinery although I don't think the caring side of it has changed, and the clients haven't changed — and that's basically what it is all about: the people. I start work at 9.00 am and usually finish around 7.00 pm. I never know

33

where the day has gone — and I've never once looked at the clock and started arranging the pencils on my desk just waiting for that last half-hour before knocking off. But I think one aspect of a vet's life that is not really apparent is the responsibility on one's shoulders; the emotional pressures put on one by the clients can be the most draining part of the job. I enjoyed my time in a mixed practice; being a country vet is a good way of life — being a small animal vet is a good job.

Liz works in a large mixed practice with six other veterinary surgeons.

I do mainly horse work, because I have always been involved with them. I had ponies as a child and looked after them myself. I also do farm animal work as necessary. There are 33 farmers who are clients of this practice, and there is only one who won't see a woman vet. If you are short there may sometimes be a problem that your arm is not long enough to feel a foetus, but I don't have any trouble at all with large animal work. My husband is doing postgraduate work on bone fractures at the moment, but eventually we will buy into a practice together or buy one from a retiring vet. We want to find a place with not too many other vets around — a friend has done well in the centre of a city. Within a year she had 7,000 clients. There are more pet owners now, especially in towns.

Chapter 2

The State Veterinary Services

Working for the Ministry does not have quite the same romantic associations as, for instance, working in a large animal practice; and that may be why there are not as many eager would-be recruits at the doors of Ministry offices as there might be. But in fact a great deal of the Ministry vet's responsibilities are concerned with farm animals, either directly or indirectly, and it has been suggested that in future the Ministry vet's involvement with animals on the farm may increase.

The Ministry is, of course, the Ministry of Agriculture, Fisheries and Food (MAFF), and the veterinary surgeons working for it are employed by the State Veterinary Service. Their responsibilities are primarily to do with food animal health, protecting the nation's flocks and herds against disease, but they are also involved with red meat and poultry meat hygiene and the improvement of farm animal welfare. There are other government organisations that are concerned with improved meat production and artificial insemination programmes.

There are three separate areas of work within the Service. The largest group are the Field Veterinary Officers who spend most of their time out visiting farms, poultry houses, slaughterhouses, ports and airports, etc. Theirs is a mainly statutory role, applying the wide range of legislation contained in the Animal Diseases Act 1981 (the Field Officer's Bible) and other legislation related to the agriculture industry; a great deal of their work is concerned with controlling notifiable diseases, such as foot and mouth, brucellosis and sheep scab, which can cause great economic damage.

The second group is based at the MAFF Veterinary Investigation Centres. The Veterinary Investigation Officers (or Veterinary Officers (VIs)) work closely with the Field Officers. They are concerned with diagnosis and control of livestock disease, both notifiable and non-notifiable, and work mainly in their centre's own laboratory, but they also visit farms at the request of the farmer's own vet to give advice on disease control.

Finally, there are staff working entirely in research at one of the Service's research laboratories.

A large number of veterinary surgeons in private practice are also employed by the Service to carry out routine work such as tuberculin testing and brucellosis sampling on herds and flocks in their area.

In England and Wales the service is linked with specialists in other fields concerned with agricultural production in the Agricultural Development and Advisory Service (ADAS) Scheme. Apart from veterinarians, ADAS advisers include agriculturists, scientists, surveyors, architects, drainage experts, etc who all work on farming problems on a local, regional or national scale.

Working for MAFF's State Veterinary Service means that you are usually doing normal office hours, and this is considered an advantage over practice work, where one might be on duty for seven days a week, 24 hours a day. However, if there is an emergency, such as an outbreak of foot and mouth, the Ministry is entitled to ask for up to three weeks of constant duty away from home, if necessary. The Ministry also expects the vets to live within a reasonable travelling distance of their work, and to be on telephone duty on a rota system.

Another advantage of Ministry work is the salary, which compares well with some, though not all, private practice work, and the possibility of promotion. And finally, there is the very important advantage that it is possible for veterinary officers to study for postgraduate courses, while being paid by the Ministry and as part of their job, under a specially appointed supervisor.

Field Veterinary Officers

Of nearly 600 veterinary surgeons in the State Veterinary Service, nearly 400 are working as field officers. There is not as much purely veterinary work in this job as in the more scientific laboratory work. The field officer's work is in many ways inspectorial because of the amount of legislation that has to be followed and in a sense he is an animal policeman, more immediately concerned with the prevention and control of animal diseases — the *raison d'etre* of the Service. He is the point of contact, as he visits slaughterhouses, knackeries, processing and cutting plants and poultry plants, as well as livestock markets and farms.

There is a lot of work in connection with diseases of poultry, including notifiable ones like Newcastle disease; hatcheries, too, are visited every quarter. There are also inspections of factories that want to export meat products; red meat hygiene and poultry meat hygiene are among the most important responsibilities. Under the Waste Food Order they carry out inspection of swill pans at the special premises licensed for the processing of waste food.

The local private veterinary surgeons, working for the Ministry on a fee paying basis and known as local veterinary inspectors, carry out most of the routine checks for diseases such as brucellosis, tuberculosis and anthrax on the farms. But field veterinary officers always do a certain percentage, partly to maintain their contact with the farmers. They are very aware that they could be thought of as 'faceless bureaucrats' at the other end of the phone, and they like to stay in touch with the farmers and be aware of what is going on. Learning to cope with people is a large part of a Ministry vet's life. Although the farmers are usually very co-operative, it may sometimes be necessary to get them to do exactly what is wanted, without seeming to bully or threaten.

So Ministry vets may go along to a farm to supervise sheep dipping, for instance, or to blood test dairy herds for brucellosis, which is done annually. If it happens that brucella is isolated, or an animal is found that is aborting

37

(brucellosis results in spontaneous abortion), the field veterinary officer advises the farmer on the best way of eradicating the disease from the herd.

Of course, field veterinary officers co-operate as much as
possible with the farmers' own vets, informing them of any
visits and giving them the opportunity of being present, as
they know the farms well. If a follow-up visit shows that a
problem still exists and appears to be insurmountable, the
field officer can call in staff from the area's Veterinary
Investigation Centre to go to the farm with him and, again,
the farmer's private vet would be informed.

A great difference between the field officers and the
private veterinary surgeons is that the former have the right
to go on to farms as part of their statutory authority. This
legal right of entry is very rarely used, and then only if
cases of notifiable disease are present or in checking on
farm animal welfare.

The subject of farm animal welfare is an important part
of the field veterinary officer's brief. Often a case may be
reported by a neighbour or the RSPCA — neither of whom
would have the same right of access to a farm. Usually a
matter of this kind is resolved quickly with the farmer, but
occasionally it is necessary to prosecute.

Another field of work is import/export inspection
which means spending time at ports and airports. Imported
meat is checked for pathogens; quarantine kennels are
checked as a matter of routine. Meat products intended for
export are checked at factories. Live animals to be exported
are also inspected; tests are carried out to satisfy the
requirements of the country of destination, and to make
sure that the animals are in a fit state to travel, as part of
the welfare responsibilities. This is an area that means
working with horses because so many are exported, and the
importers insist on specific tests; the horses or ponies may
be travelling as far as New Zealand, and may be racehorses
costing millions of pounds.

Finally, the field veterinary officer has to cope with his
or her paperwork — maybe one day a week will be taken
up in this way. However, a great many of the routine tasks

such as taking samples, inspecting markets and plants, etc, are handled by non-veterinarian technical support staff.

Veterinary Investigation Centre Staff

There are over 20 veterinary investigation centres (VICs), and their role is to provide a diagnostic and consultation service based on laboratory tests, and also to carry out local research projects.

The veterinary investigation (VI) staff are laboratory based, although they also carry out visits to farms as well. Normally tissues from diseased, or possibly diseased, animals are sent in to them by private veterinary surgeons, who have been called in by the farmer. The farmer does not deal directly with the VIC except in the case of poultry, when he may send in a carcass for post-mortem investigation.

In the laboratories the veterinary staff are able to carry out sophisticated microbiological techniques that most private veterinary surgeons would not have the facilities for in their own surgeries. Most of the animals dealt with are food animals, although they can be flexible and look at other animals as well if there is some connection with animal disease or public health, so they may in fact deal with dogs, pigeons, even budgerigars.

Normally the VIC isolates whatever the problem is, and would write back to the farmer's own vet, with a full report giving all the results of their examinations; the vet would then advise the farmer. If the VIC veterinary surgeons, in carrying out the investigation, uncover anything unusual that they have not met before and would not have associated with that particular type of environment, land or farming, they might well arrange to visit the farm.

If there is a local problem VI veterinary staff can mount small-scale local research projects. For instance, on a single farm there may be some illness that is killing the calves, and the VI staff would try to find the cause and advise the farmer on how to avoid it in the future. If there were an area problem, on perhaps five adjacent farms, with the stock losing condition and the grazing not doing as much good as it should, the VI staff would do a larger scale investigation, including analysis of the grass, to establish the cause.

VI veterinary surgeons can undertake other local research projects that are applied research, rather than relating to a specific problem on a farm or group of farms. They may wish to investigate soil content looking for mineral deficiencies, to warn the farmers of any mineral deficiency in the area. Or they may just follow a hunch that there is something that is worth while investigating.

VIC veterinary surgeons are assisted in their laboratory work by other scientific staff who carry out much of the routine work.

VICs have tended to specialise more recently in certain areas, mainly because of the cost of the equipment involved — it would be too expensive to supply each of the centres with equipment that may cost up to £15,000, so now perhaps four, or even two, centres are supplied with the equipment and they become the specialist centres for the area. One example of this specialisation is residue testing in meat. In the case of meat to be exported to certain countries, it is necessary to declare that it has passed certain tests for a minimum quantity of pesticide residue. There are only two VICs that specialise in this field, testing meat samples from all over England and Wales.

There are four VICs that have equipment for isolating viruses, and only one that specialises in brain pathology — it is obviously better to have one person in the centre working through 200 brains than 200 scattered all over the country, each working on one brain. Specialisation of this kind tends to come after veterinary surgeons have joined the Service. There is a preference for veterinary investigation rather than field posts, because it involves more purely veterinary work.

Research Staff

The third branch of the Service is the research side, the

bulk of which is at the Central Veterinary Laboratory (CVL) at Weybridge in Surrey, which is staffed, like VICs, by both vets and non-vets. There are around 60 veterinary surgeons with a lot of support staff, including scientific staff. Although it is basically a research service, staff also handle servicing work on, for instance, animals going for export, to satisfy the importing country's regulations on accepting only animals that have passed a certain number of tests and been declared free from diseases for a specified number of days before they leave the UK.

The blood and other tests that have to be carried out are usually done by the CVL and will include tests on all food animals — cattle, sheep, pigs and goats — as well as horses.

The CVL can also provide the very refined diagnostic techniques that even VICs do not have. For instance, virus isolation can be a very expensive process. Tissues are sent to the CVL for the attention of the very highly trained specialist veterinary staff — people who are already trained in one specialist area, like pathology, and whose level of expertise is higher again in one specific area in which they have specialised further.

Most of the research staff at the CVL at Weybridge specialise in a given area and work for a postgraduate qualification. They may acquire an interest in a specialist area while they are at college, maybe in poultry or sheep, or in a technique such as pathology. CVL gives them the chance to work at the subject in an applied research environment, looking at a particular problem in terms of whether the agricultural industry can be helped in some way.

All the staff are encouraged to study for higher qualifications, and they study as part of their job at the laboratory. They are normally accepted as external students of London University, although it may be with one of the other universities, and a supervisor is appointed. A scheme or work schedule is drawn up and then they work under supervision at the laboratory — so they are, in effect, paid to study. The average time for a doctorate is three years, but in fact they can take any length of time.

Postgraduate qualifications do not necessarily mean a rise in salary. Normally promotion is according to ability, but the research service is unique in that it does have a merit promotion system, if the work is of such a special nature that it merits the pay of the next higher grade.

Obviously work in a research laboratory is very much a specialist field, very scientifically orientated, and is well thought of as being something for which the veterinary surgeon has been trained at college.

Apart from the CVL at Weybridge, there are two other research laboratories, at Lasswade, Midlothian, and the Cattle Breeding Centre, Reading. The Cattle Breeding Centre investigates artificial insemination of cattle and pigs, provides a routine AI service, and carries out research on fertility and breeding.

MAFF Recruitment, Training, Promotion and Salaries

Appointments to the State Veterinary Service are made by the Civil Service Commission (address on page 107). It is possible to apply before getting a degree if you expect to qualify and become an MRCVS in the same year, but in fact the Service prefers people to have about two years' experience in an agricultural practice so that they have a knowledge of the industry and of working with farmers.

There is a short course of basic training in Civil Service procedures, and a four-week course on the general duties of the State Veterinary Service, with further periods of training according to posting. Officers can take part in local and national activities of the BVA and may occasionally attend relevant conferences at Ministry expense. After a few years in the Service there is the chance of release on full- or part-time postgraduate courses such as DVSM, Dip Bact, MSc and other courses at Ministry expense, and training is provided by the Ministry in such subjects as red meat hygiene, artificial insemination and training farmers in DIY artificial insemination. After initial training and some years of experience, veterinary officers are considered to be specialists in state veterinary medicine, and specialist posts have been created for field veterinary officers in specialist activities in poultry health, pig health, poultry meat hygiene and meat hygiene. State veterinary officers sometimes attend expenses-paid international conferences, and work connected with EEC matters or meat hygiene would often mean trips overseas. There are occasionally exchange visits, for instance involving an exchange of duties with an Australian vet, or for short study tours. Staff may also be seconded for two-year tours with the Overseas Development Administration or the Food and Agriculture Organisation (FAO) (see Chapter 6).

Salaries start at around £11,800 (1984/5 rates) for all veterinary officers. Promotion is then through divisional veterinary officer, from £16,300 to £18,600, deputy regional veterinary officer, £20,300, and regional veterinary officer, from £22,400 to £24,300. There is an additional London weighting allowance. A veterinary officer may work eight to ten years before being promoted to DVO, but many remain as veterinary officers all their lives.

Scotland

In Scotland, where the State Veterinary Service is controlled by the Department of Agriculture and Fisheries in Scotland, the veterinary investigation work is carried out not in laboratories under the control of the Ministry, but by the laboratories of the Scottish agricultural colleges. The work, though, is the same as in England and Wales with the veterinary surgeons advising the farmers and consulting with the private practice veterinary surgeons in the same way.

Northern Ireland

The work of the veterinary officers with the Department of Agriculture in Northern Ireland is basically the same as that 'over the water', but there are no VI centres as there are in England and Wales.

The work of field veterinary officers is different in that

Northern Ireland is the only part of the UK that has a land boundary with another Member State of the EEC, and so problems can arise connected with the movement of livestock across the border.

Meat inspection in Northern Ireland is centralised, unlike in England, Scotland and Wales, and therefore roughly one-third of the veterinary officers are working full time on meat inspection. There is a full-time veterinary officer in every export abattoir, every bacon factory and every poultry-slaughter plant, and he or she is responsible for hygiene and certification. The veterinary officers have a team of qualified meat inspectors working with them; these are technical officers who have done a one-year course, attending lectures by the Department's own vets, and have sat the examination for an RCVS Diploma.

The reason for this rigorous inspection of meat is that Northern Ireland is an exporter of livestock and livestock products — around 60 per cent has to be exported — and so it is essential that animal health standards are as high as possible. Import controls are also very much tighter, because an outbreak of foot and mouth or other similar diseases would be serious.

As there are no VICs, the field veterinary officers carry out some of their own investigation work.

There are two research laboratories run by the Department: the veterinary research laboratory in Stormont, Belfast, and a small satellite laboratory in Omagh. As there are no private laboratories dealing in animals in the province, the Department's staff are able to keep tabs on everything that goes through the laboratories. These research laboratories carry out the more elaborate investigations.

The Department's staff include veterinary surgeons from the rest of the UK. Salary scales are the same as MAFF's in the lower grades; but promotion and salaries are slightly different in the higher grades.

DEPARTMENT OF AGRICULTURE, DUBLIN
The Veterinary Services run by the Department of

Agriculture in Dublin cover the same areas of responsibility as those in the UK.

The veterinary inspectors in the field are involved in preventive medicine, public health, animal breeding, animal welfare, disease eradication and meat technology, and the work includes investigating disease situations and working in close contact with farmers and the veterinary profession generally. There are 27 veterinary offices throughout the country and there is an important area of work in the livestock export/import field, to prevent the spread of disease.

There are six regional laboratories and a veterinary research laboratory at Abbotsdown in County Dublin. Work at the regional laboratories is mainly of a diagnostic and advisory nature and includes field investigations and animal diseases survey work. Research includes projects related to eradication schemes, equine diseases and disease outbreaks.

A Member of the Royal College of Veterinary Surgeons would have to apply to be registered in the Register of Veterinary Surgeons for Ireland, if not already so registered. Veterinary inspectors and research officers are recruited for the Department through open competitions conducted by the Civil Service Commission, Lower Grand Canal Street, Dublin 2. All such competitions are advertised in the Irish press, usually on Wednesdays.

Other Government Agencies

The Meat and Livestock Commission

The Meat and Livestock Commission has a responsibility to improve both the quality and quantity of meat. It can become involved at every stage, from producer through abattoir, retailer and customer. It employs a few veterinary surgeons who work in all these areas, particularly the livestock improvement side. There is veterinary work in the Commission's own livestock units which are scattered throughout the country, such as pig-testing stations and bull-testing stations. These do performance testing of animals to assess their genetic merits, and then the better ones are selected for breeding. The veterinary surgeons, whose role is to give advice to the Commission and its staff, are involved in the health problems that can occur at the stations, and must prevent any infections spreading at the stations and so back to the farms. They also advise on health schemes and on the design of abattoirs. Research and development, particularly in relation to artificial insemination, is an important part of the work. Salaries are similar to MAFF scales.

Milk Marketing Board (MMB)

The MMB has 21 artificial insemination centres and about 1,000 bulls; half are Friesians but there are also other breeds, including beef breeds: Guernsey, Jersey, Shorthorn, Ayrshire, Hereford, Charollais, Limousin and Blonde d'Aquitaine. It is a legal requirement that veterinary surgeons are in attendance at these centres when semen is collected. They check on the health of the bulls, check the fertility level of the sperm and freeze it. They also provide a service of going on to farms to collect semen, freeze and store it. In addition there are veterinary surgeons at the MMB's premises in Worcester concerned with mastitis prevention and pregnancy testing.

Local Authority Work

The responsibilities of veterinary surgeons employed by local authorities are explained in Chapter 1, because the work is normally carried out on a contractual basis by people in local general practice. In England and Wales there are two towns employing full-time veterinary surgeons — Birmingham and the City of London.

In Scotland the law is different, and there are about eight local authorities with full-time veterinary surgeons, whose duties extend further than their counterparts in England and Wales. Whereas in the south the responsibilities are mainly concerned with the export of meat and the inspection of establishments such as dog breeders, boarding kennels, pet shops, riding establishments, etc, in Scotland veterinary surgeons will be responsible for all food inspection including vegetables, meat and fish. They are also concerned with sanitation and with red meat and white meat inspection at the docks, with public complaints and large food wholesalers, school and hospital meat supplies. At Edinburgh they also have the chance to teach students from the veterinary school once a week.

Salaries start at £12,000 to £15,000 for full-time veterinary surgeons, and are on a par with MAFF scales.

Home Office

The Home Office employs a small number of veterinary surgeons as inspectors; under the Cruelty to Animals Act 1876, they have the right to enter premises at any time without warning to check on the welfare of animals at research laboratories, and to inspect any animal experiment that is going on at the time to assure themselves that it is being carried out within the provisions of the Act.

Case Study

Bill is a field veterinary officer.

> I did five years in small animal and dairy practice, and then came into the Ministry because I wanted to get married and have a family. I was in field jobs in two separate counties, and then worked at Birkenhead in connection with the import of animals from Ireland. Then I worked at the head office at Tolworth for five years, and was able to go all over the world — China, America and several European countries. I probably travelled more than most people; they were mostly visits concerned with the welfare of animals being exported by air, sea, road, rail and hovercraft (they've all got special problems). I was very busy at Tolworth, working on animal welfare countrywide as well as abroad. At the same time I did a doctorate on farm control of animal welfare. It was a private venture but I was helped considerably by the Ministry.

Chapter 3
Teaching and Research

Like human medicine, veterinary medicine involves a great deal of scientific training and knowledge, as well as caring. Graduates from veterinary school who have decided they enjoy the purely scientific side of the work and are interested in pursuing some special scientific interest will find that there are several areas open to them for continuing with that part of their training.

Some graduates work in practice for a while and decide that the long hours do not suit them, or that they prefer to work in a field in which they can be more in control of their own work, as they are when doing a research project. Research may also appeal to women as a long-term plan, because they might later be able to find a job with hours that fit more easily into family life than working in practice. The veterinary profession, as one research worker put it, is a very good profession to get into: if you have a veterinary degree there is a wide choice open to you.

Opportunities for research exist in institutes such as those run under the auspices of the Agricultural and Food Research Council or Medical Research Council, the Animal Health Trust (which is a charity), at Ministry of Agriculture laboratories, see Chapter 2, in private research centres and large pharmaceutical companies. There is also a lot of research at the universities, done by the teaching staff because university funding is now very much dependent on research success, and so taking on someone who is not going to produce a reasonable volume of research would be termed counter-productive.

For work in teaching or research, the veterinary graduate

would normally also need to have completed a postgraduate course leading to a PhD. This is usually at least a three-year course and is purely research work, and gained by thesis — you undertake a piece of original research, write it up and present a thesis and also undergo a short oral examination before a board of specialists in that field. As postgraduate work involves finding grants both to finance the student's personal living expenses and the research work itself, a job in which you can take a PhD while being paid by the employer is very helpful. It will mean that the three years can stretch out to as many as 12. This situation can exist in MAFF laboratories, AFRC institutes and occasionally in universities, but not in all commercial companies.

An MSc is also a useful qualification when looking for research or teaching work. Generally speaking it is a one-year course for which there is a syllabus set by a university, and it is usually awarded for a combination of examination and the preparation of a small thesis; it involves a small area of research and a small paper on that research. Occasionally there is a part-time MSc, which is taken over two years.

Some veterinary students can exercise the option of intercalating a year in the middle of their university course and taking a BSc before the final clinical years. There is a variety of courses in subjects such as anatomy, biochemistry, pharmacology and physiology. This would be taken at other schools within the university. This is a most valuable prelude to a research career because it is exactly the training that pure scientists receive and it is much more concerned with looking at a few subjects in detail, unlike most of the veterinary courses in which the student needs to grasp a tremendous variety of subject matter rather than delving in depth into tiny areas. Many students take the BSc as it is a very useful addition to their course, and could also be attractive to a general practice.

Teaching

Before taking up a teaching position, a veterinary graduate

would do either or both of the following: he or she would do a PhD course either at a university — although not necessarily in a veterinary department — or at a research institute, supervised from a university, or he or she would go into practice for a year or two to gain experience. It is possible to do a PhD while teaching, although it is difficult because teaching is a full-time job and it is not easy to find enough time for the extra work. Normally the graduate arranges for postgraduate funding through a senior member of staff who approaches a body such as the Agricultural and Food Research Council or the Wellcome Trust for finance, for both the research and to support the student during the three years needed to get a PhD.

Teachers who will be lecturing in the clinical departments will very often have spent some time in practice — although it can be difficult to give up the higher standard of living that practice gives, compared with academic salaries. It is not so essential for non-clinical teaching staff to have experience in practice.

At some veterinary schools a new idea is catching on from the USA. Called a 'residency programme', it provides graduates with one to three years of specialist clinical postgraduate training rather as a doctor might have in an NHS hospital if he or she wanted to become, say, a neurologist or psychiatrist. This is an excellent way for young vets who want to end up teaching in clinical departments to acquire a very high level of specialist training, not only from the clinical point of view but also in research skills. It is hoped that this will produce more highly trained young veterinary teachers. The scheme is run by the universities, but provided by a private trust interested in education that wants to close the gap between the procedures of postgraduate training that has existed up to now between human and veterinary medical students.

Occasionally veterinary surgeons may decide that they would like to change after a considerable time spent in a career in industry or general practice, and move into university teaching. They may even have owned a private practice and feel they have a vocation for teaching and would like to put the benefit of maybe 10 or 15 years' experience into the academic world. Although they would enter the teaching profession at a high level, as reader or professor, it does mean that they would certainly be taking a tremendous cut in salary.

New university teachers are subject to a three-year probationary period and during that time they must demonstrate not only that they are capable of teaching the students effectively, but also that they have defined some area of research and begun work on it; in a clinical department they would have had to build up a small area of work in which they could specialise, and so be able to give expert advice on referral cases (see below). At the end of the three years most teaching staff are confirmed in their appointment but, if they have failed to come up to scratch, their appointment would be terminated at the end of the three-year period.

Most teaching is done by lectures and practical instruction. The pre-clinical years, including subjects such as anatomy and pathology, are the ones in which research by the teaching staff is necessary. They have freedom to do whatever research they like, but the research is not funded by the University Grants Committee (UGC), and so it is necessary to look to one of the funding bodies for any necessary finance.

The clinical years involve teaching the students in small groups, with animals. Veterinary schools are similar to medical schools in that not only do they have the responsibility to teach the students and conduct research, but they also see referral cases as part of the work. These are cases for specialists in various fields that are referred, in the case of veterinary school, to the veterinary hospital of the university via the veterinary surgeon in practice, to solve a problem that has defied him or her or to use techniques that he or she may not have access to. There are also free clinics at the universities, to provide the students with a flow of ordinary cases from the locality so that they can become used to examining cats and dogs, etc, diagnosing disease, talking to the owner about it and learning how to

51

treat the condition — all experience for practice work.

Large animal teaching takes place on farms or in practices owned by the college in agricultural areas outside the university town. An advantage of clinical work within a university is that there is the chance to use up-to-date diagnostic and surgical equipment that is not available to the general practitioner.

University research is less pressurised than full-time research in that if the teachers' research hits a rough patch, even for a year, they are tided over the setback by the fact that there is a much broader range of activities that they are involved in, although of course they must not slacken up on the research programme; equally there is the stimulus, even in research, of being continuously questioned by students, who can have extremely searching queries. On the other hand, in a research institute there are none of the distractions of a university term.

For the students themselves, it is more difficult to do research while at university, because a lot of research is covered by legislation which precludes them from acting even as helpers until they are licensed. They can, however, help in minor capacities under supervision, and in some areas of the course they would do mini-research projects like comparing blood samples with productivity in cows.

Houseman

The post of houseman is a junior one in a clinical department, and basically it provides a training in clinical work in surgery or medicine. The houseman will have recently qualified and helps in running the veterinary hospital's clinic; it gives the chance of getting relevant experience for practice or in the clinical department of a university and would help anyone wanting to specialise in X-raying or anaesthesia, or medicine or surgery, and at the same time look for a junior post in a university department.

Other Teaching Posts

Some teaching in universities is done on a part-time basis by staff in research institutes. General practitioners take a share in teaching at the agricultural colleges, also on a part-time basis — they do not employ veterinary surgeons as full-time teaching staff.

Salaries

Salary scales for academic staff are unfortunately among the lowest in the veterinary profession. They start at around £7,520 for assistant lecturer and lecturer and continue up to £14,925. Senior lecturer/reader level is £14,135 to £17,705 and Professor £18,070 (average: £21,235). Assistant lecturers and lecturers aged 27 years or over start at £8,920 (1984 rates).

Research

The fundamental difference between teaching and research in an institute or other laboratory is that 100 per cent of your time will be spent in research. Most days you would not even see a live animal. For people who are tremendously motivated towards research, who have perhaps become interested in some particular field while at university, and who are blessed with the ability to come up regularly with subjects for research work that are worth doing, this type of career is very satisfying. It calls for a particular type of temperament that combines imagination with an ability to keep slogging away at routine work, and cope with frustration — even the finest research workers have periods when things are not running the way they would want. Someone with a research mentality, who is interested in physiology or disease processes in certain areas, would go where the interest is, and it would not matter to him or her whether the work was in MAFF, an institute or industrial research — although the pressures would probably be greater in industrial research.

An aspect of research that could be overlooked is the tropical side. Britain has a long tradition in tropical veterinary medicine; specialisation in this field can lead to doing work in the developing countries that could not be carried out in the UK.

Agricultural and Food Research Council (AFRC)

Scientists specialising in all kinds of subjects work for the Agricultural and Food Research Service, which is run by the Agricultural and Food Research Council (AFRC), formerly known as the Agricultural Research Council. The Council was set up to oversee the independent institutes that developed in the 1930s, to make sure that research efforts were not duplicated in some areas and neglected in others. There are now about 38 institutes and units around the country. Some are administered directly by the AFRC and others are state aided, and the research is overseen by the AFRC whereas the staff are employed by the institutes and so there is a degree of independence. A list of the institutes and units and a full summary of the work they do is available from the AFRC (address on page 107). Not all of them employ veterinary surgeons, and some have only one on the staff.

The institutes are all concerned with increasing productivity and improving quality, and the veterinary surgeons deal only with farm animals and their diseases. An advantage for the research worker is that he or she is a member of a team all of whom will be working on the same problem, rather than working in isolation. It is very stimulating to be able to exchange ideas with other scientists and to co-operate with them in the work. There is also the chance to use the latest laboratory equipment. There are technical assistants to help with routine tasks and specialists to advise on subjects such as statistical analysis of research results.

Some of the institutes concentrate only on cattle or sheep, others on poultry or pigs. It is not part of the Agricultural and Food Research Council's responsibilities to work on horses but the Animal Virus Research Institute (based in Pirbright) has undertaken contract work for the Horserace Betting Levy Board (HBLB). The institutes concentrate on the elimination or reduction of animal diseases and some of their work takes them out into the field. Usually the veterinary surgeon is dealing with problems as they arise, often as a result of changes in the management of animals; for as greater numbers of animals are kept on farms, the intensification of livestock means that there are more animals per metre, and therefore diseases can arise that have not been a problem before, or they can arise in greater proportion and become more significant than they have been before.

The institutes have a fairly wide remit and can be concerned with the whole of the UK, if the work that they are doing is applicable. There are regional differences in disease, and a particular disease may be less important in one area than another, and so an institute may be primarily concerned with local problems, but as in the whole of the UK the same diseases generally occur, their work can be of benefit nationally.

Institutes in Scotland will also do veterinary investigation work for the Ministry, collaborating with the Veterinary Investigation Service. If a farmer has a disease problem, and his vet contacts the VI service, they may pass material on to one of the institutes for further investigation. If necessary the institute will not only give a diagnosis, but also undertake research to find the cause of the problem, how it arose and how to combat it.

Some of the veterinary surgeons working with the Agricultural Research Service have worked in practice first, and then decided they wanted to take up research. This may be because they became disillusioned with the routine of practice, or because they developed a particular interest in a specific type of work. They may have become interested in biochemistry and in the metabolic problems that follow with such diseases as milk fever; and so they decide they would like to investigate these problems to a greater depth. Other people decide on research while they are at college.

The ARS would normally expect a veterinary surgeon to have a PhD, but they may take on someone with particular expertise in one special area who has perhaps a BSc in biochemistry, or has done a one- or two-year postgraduate course in a subject such as microbiology for an MSc. If there is a vacancy for such people within the ARS, and they have been taken on, it is possible for them to work for a higher degree and get a PhD within the Service. Staff were once encouraged to move on every five years or so, so that they could widen their training and experience, but unfortunately, because of the recent cutbacks in funding for posts both in the ARS and the universities, it is now more difficult to move easily from one job to another, because of the lack of openings. Some may go back into practice, although this can be difficult if they are out of touch with practice work; the majority stay in research, or may go into the universities, to pharmaceutical firms, or occasionally to university posts abroad — remaining in some kind of academic life.

Salary is at the same scale as in the Ministry of Agriculture's State Veterinary Service (see page 43). Staff are taken on as veterinary research officers (VROs) and are promoted to principal veterinary research officers (PVROs). The higher grades are mainly used in the management and organisation of research, and are dependent on the existence of vacancies. It is possible to be promoted eventually to director of an institute or, occasionally, to be promoted on merit, so that outstanding scientists can continue to work without having to undertake administrative responsibilities.

As well as offering postgraduate studentships, the AFRC also makes short-term grants to universities to support promising new lines of research.

The AFRC and State-Aided Institutes that do Veterinary Work

Animal Breeding Research Organisation, King's Buildings, West Mains Road, Edinburgh EH9 3JQ. The work is concerned with research on the genetics of farm animals, with livestock based on experimental farms and laboratory studies. The animals being studied are cattle, pigs and sheep and subjects under research are lean meat production, aspects of immunogenetics, fertilisation and the survival and development of embryos. The Organisation liaises with the Meat and Livestock Commission and Milk Marketing Board and gives advice to animal breeders.

Institute of Animal Physiology, Babraham, Cambridge CB2 4AT. The Institute is concerned with improved animal production and consists of two farms and groups of laboratories and surgeries at Babraham and Girton. It includes the Monoclonal Antibody Centre as well as departments of behavioural physiology and neuroendocrinology.

Institute for Research on Animal Diseases, Compton, Newbury, Berkshire RG16 0NN. The Institute studies economically important diseases of farm animals, particularly cattle and pigs. Cattle, sheep and pigs are bred at the Institute, and much of the food for them is also grown on the Institute's farms. The Institute contains six research departments and sections: biochemistry, immunology, microbiology, pathology, clinical medicine and surgery section as well as a statistics section.

Poultry Research Centre, Roslin, Midlothian EH25 9PS. The Centre is eight miles south of Edinburgh. Research is aimed at increasing the biological efficiency of poultry production and maintaining and improving poultry welfare and is concerned with physiology, metabolism, nutrition, environment, behaviour, genetics, and metabolic pathology.

Animal Virus Research Institute, Pirbright, Woking, Surrey GU24 0NF. Work on foot and mouth disease was started at Pirbright as long ago as 1924 and has continued ever since. The Institute is the world reference laboratory for foot and mouth disease and is responsible for typing and classifying the virus as it occurs overseas as well as in Britain. It is also researching into the preparation of foot and mouth vaccine, to make it easier to use in field conditions overseas. The Institute was also involved in the detection of swine vesicular disease in 1972 and its work on other viruses includes rabies, African swine fever, African horse sickness and bluetongue, to establish diagnostic facilities in case the diseases were likely to be brought into the UK.

Grassland Research Institute, Hurley, Maidenhead, Berkshire SL6 5LR. Research is undertaken on grass and forage, and the animals on the Institute's farm are dairy cows, beef cattle and sheep. There is a veterinary unit and work is done on animal nutrition and production. The Grassland Veterinary Research Group investigates the causes and prevention of animal disorders associated with legumes and with mineral deficiencies.

Houghton Poultry Research Station, Houghton, Huntingdon, Cambridgeshire PE17 2DA. The Station investigates the causes and control of avian diseases, particularly those causing the most serious economic loss to the poultry industry, such as infectious bronchitis and bacterial infections (particularly salmonella) and studies interrelated problems in the fields of biochemistry and physiology. The Station staff do some teaching of veterinary students at Cambridge University and contribute to postgraduate and undergraduate courses for the Royal Veterinary College, London. Suitably qualified staff and students are usually able to register for courses for higher degrees.

National Institute for Research in Dairying, Shinfield, Reading, Berkshire RG2 9AT. The Institute's animals are mainly dairy cattle, of course, but there is also work on pigs, concerned with the use in their diet of dairy by-products. The programmes generally are involved with such subjects as feeding, mastitis, reproduction and nutrition.

Hill Farming Research Organisation, Bush Estate, Penicuik, Midlothian EH26 0PY. The work of the Organisation is designed to apply to hill farming throughout the UK and some of the research work involves collaboration with other institutes that specialise in soils and animal breeding and nutrition and animal diseases. The animals studied are both sheep and cattle in four departments: animal production, animal nutrition, grazing ecology and plants and soils.

Moredun Institute (ADRA), 408 Gilmerton Road, Edinburgh

EH17 7JH. The Moredun has more veterinary surgeons on the staff than the other AFRC institutes and units. A number of senior staff are recognised as members of the academic staff of the University of Edinburgh and the Institute is approved for postgraduate training and for registration for higher degrees. They concentrate essentially on cattle and sheep and the work is principally to investigate the causes of diseases in farm livestock and to formulate methods of prevention; another important area of work is towards increasing livestock productivity. The Institute collaborates with other institutes, such as the Animal Breeding Research Station and the Hill Farming Research Organisation. The microbiology and pathology departments are concerned with microbial infections that cause losses in animal production; the biochemistry department, which includes a radio-isotope section, works on production diseases, and the parasitology department studies parasitic worms and host-parasite relationships. The department of physiology has studied death in lambs immediately after birth and has devised methods of resuscitating lambs which have been exposed to cold, wet conditions and starvation.

Rowett Research Institute, Bucksburn, Aberdeen AB2 9SB. The Institute's work relates to the nutrition of all farm livestock, and balances the basic studies of the biological processes involved in animal production and the applied aspects of feeding and management of animals. Some aspects of the work are of relevance to the nutrition of man. The Institute shares in the teaching of Aberdeen University's MSc degree course in animal nutrition.

Although all the institutes and units mentioned do have veterinary surgeons on the staff, the numbers are not great. However, the descriptions give an idea of the type of work done in research laboratories, and of the many scientific avenues explored with the purpose of increasing food and livestock production, and protecting livestock from disease.

Medical Research Council (MRC)

The MRC has veterinary surgeons on its staff, although the Council is concerned with diseases and other medical conditions in humans, not animals. Some of the veterinary surgeons are engaged in research work with the Council, and their work gives them the chance of collaborating in the biomedical field with other scientists and medical specialists; other veterinary surgeons are in charge of laboratory animals or experimental surgical facilities.

The work is carried on at the Council's research establishments, some attached to universities and some to hospitals. Research subjects include the genetic nature of transplants, microsurgery, immunology, transplant rejection; there are also veterinary surgeons working in the laboratories concerned with animal welfare in the laboratories, and laboratory animal husbandry.

Vacancies are usually advertised in scientific journals and newspapers. There is no central recruitment through the Council's head office, but people can apply to individual units to ask if there is a vacancy (apply to the Director). Leaflets giving details of MRC careers and a list of the establishments are available from the MRC head office (address on page 108). More detailed information about the type of work done in each establishment is given in the Medical Research Council's Handbook, which should be in the reference section of public libraries, or available from HMSO or the MRC, price £5.50 including p & p.

Recruitment and Salaries

The MRC normally expects its non-clinical (ie non-medical) staff to have done a year in practice or to have a PhD from a veterinary school, or relevant experience. There are two types of appointment: the short-term appointments are normally for three to five years and are intended for those who have just obtained their PhD or equivalent and who are looking for further experience in full-time research; career appointments are for more experienced scientists and are expected to be permanent, until retirement age. This second type of employment can involve changes in field of work, and also in the place of work (some of the MRC's staff work overseas).

Salaries are related to salaries in universities and other bodies in closely related fields, and start at £7,520 to £11,205 with London allowance (1985 scale). There is, of course, the possibility of promotion for senior staff, with salaries up to £23,650 for special appointments.

Animal Health Trust

The Trust is a charity, with income derived from donations, fund-raising events and deeds of covenant, plus grants for specific research projects and the professional services the Trust provides for the veterinary profession. The work is with horses and domestic animals — not with food animals. However, there is a limited number of research scholarships and fellowships awarded by the Trust for the study of diseases in farm animals, fish and poultry, and the work for these is carried out at other suitable institutes in the UK.

The Trust operates from two centres at Newmarket in Suffolk. They are the Equine Research Station at Balaton Lodge, and the Small Animals Centre at Lanwades Park.

Balaton Lodge has several units. The immunology unit blood-types thoroughbred horses, Shires, Arabs and other breeds for the General Stud Book. The pathology unit investigates horses, especially problems affecting reproduction in mares and diseases of foals and yearlings, and also provides services to veterinary surgeons in practice; some of the work they do is also in collaboration with doctors and other specialists in human medicine. The clinical unit has a powerful X-ray machine to help in the diagnosis of back and other orthopaedic conditions in horses, and the unit also has diagnostic laboratories. The laboratories test samples sent in by practices to diagnose illnesses in dogs and cats, as well as horses. Thousands of samples are handled each year and the laboratories are semi-automated and computerised. A service is also provided to racehorse trainers, through their veterinary surgeons, to check on the blood of horses in training — this can give early warning of the possibility of over-training, stress and infections.

Lanwades Park specialises in small animals. An important unit is the ophthalmology unit which handles cases of eye problems in pedigree dogs, cats and horses, sent to the unit by veterinary surgeons for surgery and treatment. Some of the cases recently have included a gorilla, a cheetah, a snow leopard and a Canadian timber wolf, and the staff also advise the dog breeding societies about breed standards, in an effort to reduce some of the hereditary eye abnormalities. The unit provides a regular service to the Guide Dogs for the Blind Association. The bacteriology unit carries out research as well as providing a back-up service to the veterinary practices, for animals sent in with problems that can range from respiratory problems in racehorses to dogs with ear trouble. The virology unit also looks into respiratory problems in horses and assists in the development of new types of vaccine, some of which involve genetic engineering. A new unit is the oncology unit, dealing with tumours of all kinds in dogs and cats. Another part of the Small Animals Centre is the duck unit.

The work of the Trust is interesting in that it deals with live animals and provides treatment for which it has now established a world-wide reputation. Unfortunately for some of the research projects, funding can run out, so that the projects have to be wound up.

Recruitment and Salaries

Salaries are linked to university scales. Veterinary graduates who are taken on usually have two to three years' experience in practice or other work, and can study for higher degrees while working with the Trust.

Research Centres and Pharmaceutical Companies

Veterinary surgeons work for the large pharmaceutical (drugs) companies in various fields, not all of them to do with research. And they are also employed by smaller research laboratories that operate on a contract basis, evaluating the safety of pharmaceutical products, pesticides and industrial chemicals.

In the research departments of the large companies they work alongside biologists, doctors and pharmacologists in the research and development of drugs, vaccines and anti-sera that will be used by either humans or animals. Because the veterinary market is a relatively small one, the pharmaceutical companies hope that the drugs they produce will have a wide application, and not many of the drugs are produced specifically with animals in mind. Veterinary surgeons working alongside the other scientists try to apply the drugs being developed to veterinary uses. They are involved both in the basic stages of the research and in the more applied stages. Those more specifically concerned with veterinary products are involved nearer the end of the development stage, adapting the products to a more specifically veterinary application. For instance, products designed to deal with such things as worms, fleas, ticks and lice have to be presented in special compounds or formulations for veterinary use — it is not always easy to get a horse to take a pill, for instance, and it is much better to develop a special formulation of paste that the animal will accept more easily.

Basic development work done behind the scenes involves, for instance, the development of vaccines; the research workers in the laboratories have to grow the organism, produce the particular part of the organism that is going to be used for the vaccine or, if it is a live vaccine, find a type of organism that is no longer disease-producing. Or they have to isolate the substances that the organism produces that are going to form the basis of the vaccine — all very fundamental scientific work. Other types of work include producing substances that can aid diagnosis in laboratories, to help in the identification of a certain infection in an animal, or developing techniques for the identification of other changes in the animal.

An important role for veterinary surgeons in research is

that of toxicological pathology. There are a large number doing this work now because of the government requirement both of the UK and the USA that drugs and other chemicals that come into contact with the public should be tested to check whether they are poisonous or not. A lot of evidence has to be produced when there is a new drug ready to be launched on the market, to prove that the drug is safe. And so these drugs are tested in laboratory animals: mice, dogs and primates. All the organs of all the animals that have been dosed are required to be examined by pathologists both at post-mortem and by microscopic examination afterwards. Toxicologists are involved at every stage of the development of new drugs, from basic research onwards, because obviously if the product does turn out to be toxic there is no point in proceeding with it. Although the job has been described as less interesting than research, because 'you end up looking at a lot of normal histology of normal rats, which is rather boring', the pay is better than at research institutes.

Other areas of work in pharmaceutical companies — clinical trials, marketing and advisory — are described in Chapter 4.

Qualifications and Salaries

Research work is becoming increasingly specialised and there is much greater specialisation now in all fields of biomedical research, particularly in toxicology. Most people joining a pharmaceutical company will have done a PhD after graduating from veterinary school, or gained further experience working in a laboratory in a research institute or with MAFF, or if they have answered an advertisement for a post that calls for specialised training, may have gained that experience with another pharmaceutical company (there is much more opportunity for moving around between jobs in industry than there is in other research fields). However, the large companies and private research centres will also give on-the-job training and the chance of working with experienced specialists,

and there can also be opportunities for further education
leading to higher academic and professional qualifications.

Salaries depend on qualifications and experience. The
general picture is that it is not as good as working in practice, better than at a university; a graduate with four or
five years' experience would perhaps receive around
£14,000 — about the same as an assistant in practice at that
stage, but not comparable with a partnership. Obviously if
a company is looking for someone with specialised knowledge they would be prepared to pay reasonably for that
specialised knowledge.

Research Abroad

There are opportunities for working in laboratories abroad
with organisations like the Overseas Development Administration, whose work is described in Chapter 6, as well as
for the government services of individual countries. Advertisements for these posts appear in the *Veterinary Record*.

Postgraduate Research and Grants

The Royal College of Veterinary Surgeons' handbook,
'A Career as a Veterinary Surgeon', lists the postgraduate
training facilities at universities that have veterinary schools
in the UK and the Republic of Ireland, together with other
postgraduate qualifications open to veterinary graduates
including diplomas of the RCVS and diplomas and degrees
offered by universities other than by the veterinary schools
in the UK and Ireland, which are open to veterinary graduates. Postgraduate awards and grants are available for
veterinary graduates and in the veterinary field from such
bodies as the Wellcome Trust, the ODA, AFRC, Animal
Health Trust, Horserace Betting Levy Board, etc. The
booklet provides a full list of all the grant-awarding bodies.

Case Studies

David works in a research institute.

> I went to Edinburgh·University and did one year in a large
> animal practice in Snowdonia. My family were all in veter-

inary surgery (I'm the sixth generation) and two were professors at Edinburgh University, so it was natural for me to think of going into research. I found that in large animal practice you are basically doing what other people — the farmers — require you to do; sometimes at 3.00 am — whereas in research you are more in charge of your own day. I was interested in infectious diseases and was very lucky to be able to find a post in a research institute — the Moredun. You can find that the longer you leave it, the more difficult it is to compete with recent graduates. Since I started it has become almost impossible for me to go back into university life because I would have to take a massive cut in salary.

Some of my time here is spent doing consultancy diagnosis for the Veterinary Investigation Service. One of my specialties is brain pathology: neuropathology. There's an awful lot of brain disease about. A colleague and I cover the whole of Scotland and do some consultancy work for England and Wales. I work with the microscope for a while every afternoon and decide from the slide what disease each particular sheep has. It's computerised now, so I punch my report into the terminal, press a button and a letter is typed out with all the details along with my report, and it signs itself for me; and that goes off to the Veterinary Investigation Centre. We don't investigate disease outbreaks, but we are research specialists and have equipment that the VIC can't afford. The Centre receives our report, talks to the farm and the vet and collates all the information.

A job at a VIC suits someone who doesn't want to specialise and who likes a general life. They can get out and about in the car and live in the country. In my type of job I very rarely get out.

We have other genuine research projects such as one at the moment in which we are working on a mystery agent that is killing cattle and red deer; we don't know the cause yet. It is not a great plague that is sweeping the country — no one has heard about it in the trade — but it is a problem and causes a most unpleasant type of disease for which there is no cure. In that case we do get out and about to fetch animals in that are very poorly, and it allows us to get some specimens for our work. We've travelled a lot of Scotland and even been down to Northampton to pick up a carcass. It's a very strange and interesting disease and we think it is caused by a virus — it seems to fall halfway between a virus and certain forms of cancer. I work on that as a pathologist in close collaboration with another veterinary surgeon, who's a virologist. I look down the microscope at dead tissue, sliced very thin and stained up, and he spends all his time in another room culturing cells — taking tissue cultures and nurturing them seven days a week.

I did my doctorate at the Institute; it was allowed because it was Institute work and I was one of the fortunate few — and was being paid a salary. My head of department was my supervisor here. I had to work harder to do it, but that was a small price to pay.

Paul works for the MRC.

I did a year in practice as a houseman at Bristol Veterinary School before starting with the MRC. I got the job by answering an advertisement. We are looking at the problems of low birthweight babies and babies that are too small for their age. We have a paediatrician working with us and are looking at ways of improving their medical treatment. We started off looking at runt animals because we thought they might have the same problems as the babies, checking with the hand-rearing book. We look at the effects of clinical treatment and the paediatrician compares the effects of treatment on the babies in the special-care units. I enjoy working on a project that has a fairly clear outcome.

Chapter 4

Commercial Companies, Zoos and the Royal Army Veterinary Corps

Pharmaceutical Companies

The research side of the work in drugs companies has been covered in Chapter 3, but these companies employ veterinary surgeons in many other capacities that are connected with the development of the drug through to marketing and advising farmers and veterinary surgeons in general practice on their use.

For somebody who enjoys being part of a large organisation, with none of the pressures of running a business that being in practice involves, and who would prefer to work fewer hours, this type of job can seem preferable to being a 24-hour all-weather vet. For married women it is easier to go back into a job with a large company than it is into practice, and there are also good chances of promotion for the right people.

However, better hours are not true of every job, and working for a pharmaceutical company can mean spending periods abroad, even for research workers; while marketing in any business can involve a great deal of time on the road.

Linked with the basic research staff are veterinary surgeons involved in the clinical or field trials of the new products. This is done after the drug has been tested in the laboratories and involves veterinary products only. It basically means testing to see if it does actually work on the animals, as it should, and doing final trials on the animals before it is released on to the market. This is done on farms, and means making arrangements with the farmer, and then getting the results. Sometimes conducting field trials with new products needs to be done on quite a large scale and, depending on the product, may mean co-operating with the Ministry of Agriculture. Compared with research work it does give the veterinary surgeon the chance to work with and treat live animals.

Clinical, or field, trials work may be carried out overseas as well as in the UK. If a new insecticide, for instance, is developed, it is necessary to know whether it works not only against ticks in cattle in the UK but also in other countries such as Australia, Africa and South America to make sure it does not produce undesirable effects in cattle abroad. It may be perfectly all right to use on cattle in Surrey, and no use at all in Arizona. Or it may be necessary to test something at a time of the year when the problem does not occur in this country. If a product is for export, the country concerned will often require local trials before they will license its sale. Many of the large companies are large exporters and need veterinary surgeons to work overseas permanently to deal with technical servicing and promotional work.

Technical servicing or technical support backs up the marketing side of the company. There the veterinary surgeons give advice both to the product users and to the sales staff. It means going to meetings with veterinary surgeons, advising on the technicalities of the product being marketed, seeing farmers and wholesalers who provide products of all kinds, including drugs, to farmers. There are often scientific meetings involving veterinary surgeons in practice or business meetings involving farmers to discuss products, or perhaps a specific disease problem. This work also involves answering any technical queries, dealing with any complaints (troubleshooting, in other words) and advising marketing staff on the correct strategy to apply with regard to promotions. For example, a marketing man might need guidance on avoiding making some promotional ploy which was clinically undesirable or even illegal.

Other problems may crop up if an animal receives a drug but dies unexpectedly, or an animal has been vaccinated but has still got the disease, or there may be a particularly difficult outbreak of a disease on a farm where they think they might be able to use the product but, because it is abnormal, they need advice on how to use it to the best effect. Such health problems may involve going out into the field, collecting samples, liaison with laboratory research people, post-mortem examination, and discussions with the farmer's own veterinary surgeon.

It is also possible for a veterinary surgeon to work on the sales side of the company full time, rather than in the technical support for the sales department, and also to move up into senior management and administration.

Most of the large pharmaceutical companies have veterinary surgeons in several countries overseas, because they are usually multi-national organisations. Some are specifically hired to work abroad.

Qualifications and Salaries

Work involving field trials and technical servicing would require some practical experience, but not necessarily a postgraduate qualification. The clinical skills needed anyway form part of the university training programme, and further training would come from practice work. The more broadly based the practical experience, the better. Very few graduates would go straight from college into a commercial company; normally they go into practice for three to five years, see a post advertised for somebody to carry out some form of drug trials with a pharmaceutical company, apply for it and, with luck, are successful because of their experience. Very often having the right temperament is more important than the experience.

For work abroad, a commercial company would usually be looking for someone with experience abroad — if they want to test something in Africa, for instance, they need somebody who knows about African conditions and can test a new compound in those conditions — so UK experience may be of less use. Often those working abroad will have started with an organisation like Voluntary Service Overseas (VSO), and gone into an Overseas Development

Administration (ODA) job or worked for an overseas government for a while; they could have had a job in the Kenyan government, for example, and then taken a job with a company such as the Wellcome Foundation in that country, either working in a laboratory or in the field. Someone who has been working on a laboratory-based ODA project in Kenya might also move into a Wellcome laboratory there when the project ended, or be sent by Wellcome to another country such as Australia.

As always, salaries, even in senior posts, are quoted as not being as much as a partner would receive in a successful practice, but of course there is not the up-front commitment of having to buy into a practice. As in the area of research, one might expect to go in at around £14,000, but of course this is a highly competitive area and would be an individual matter. When a man or woman is interviewed the company has to decide whether he or she can provide a quality that the company needs and have the particular attributes wanted at the time — and even have a particular personality that fits in with what is wanted. The right people get more pay, and there is anyway the chance of promotion. They are not necessarily expected to stay in the same job, and there may be opportunities to move around within the framework of the company.

Laboratory Animal Houses

The care and responsibility for the health status of animal houses in both pharmaceutical companies and universities are increasingly being met by veterinary surgeons. Although the subject of laboratory animals is a sensitive one, most 'middle of the road' people concerned about animal welfare would like to see the conditions under which experimental animals are kept in responsible hands, and the profession, too, would like to see a professional doing that job. Proposed new legislation will require the facilities to have a nominated veterinary surgeon in charge, and already individuals wishing to carry out experimental research using animals must be licensed by the Home Office and have a licence that specifically covers them for the things they wish to do.

Another aspect of laboratory animal work is that if one has the expense of keeping a number of animals, including primates which are very valuable animals, it is important to have a veterinary surgeon responsible for the animal house facilities.

Veterinary surgeons work full time or part time as animal house directors or curators. Part-time curators may also be doing research work, perhaps related to toxicology or pathology, either in a university department or within the research department of a pharmaceutical company. They are responsible for the management, in the widest sense of the term, of the facilities housing animals for experimental work. They are responsible for the day-to-day running of the animal house (with the help of technicians), making policy decisions on how the facility should be run and training the technicians. They must have an understanding of the disease and welfare aspects of animals and also have an understanding of what the animals are being used for — making ethical judgements in terms of advising what is a suitable model for a particular study, whether a procedure is likely to be painful for an animal, what anaesthetics to use during surgery and surgical techniques. (There are veterinary surgeons assisting in heart transplant surgery.) The curator may also teach research workers about surgical techniques. He or she will also need to know about the role of disease in the animal facilities, and this may involve advice on the design of the units, and suitability for the different species.

It is a job which means using the whole of a veterinary training and applying it to a group of animals that are no different from any others except for the purpose for which they are there.

The role of the curator or director is broadly the same whether it is in a university or a pharmaceutical company. Universities are now tending to centralise their animal house facilities and this includes those that do not have a veterinary school attached, as the facilities will be used by medical schools and other departments as well. The area is an expanding one — the Laboratory Animals Group of the British Veterinary Association has about 180 members, although not all of them are working full time. It is a relatively new area of specialisation, with an increase of interest because of new postgraduate training and because the new legislation will increase the number of jobs. Postgraduate courses are approved by the Royal College, some universities, and by the BVA group, which runs weekend courses in laboratory animal management.

Salaries are variable. The curators of university animal houses are usually paid on the scale of academic other related staff (grade III): £14,135 to £17,705. They would be expected to have extensive experience in the production and care of laboratory animals and, as well as their veterinary degree, hold a higher degree in a relevant field of study, or have other appropriate qualifications and experience.

Directors of animal houses in pharmaceutical companies would tend to have a higher salary. An advantage of this work is that it gives the opportunity to carry out research.

Working in a Zoo

In the UK

The idea of working with zoo animals is a very attractive one — the secretary of the BVA's zoological society gets many letters from graduates hoping to do this kind of job. But unfortunately, in the UK in particular, the field is very limited for vets who qualify and then wish to specialise in zoo medicine or surgery. There are no longer many zoos, and with the Zoo Licensing Act now in force, some of the smaller zoos are being forced to close down. It seems likely that there will be a polarisation of interest into the larger zoo complexes and it will be in these zoo complexes that the opportunities for employment will be greatest in the UK.

The particular ones in Britain are the London Zoological Society, and the universities which are associated with zoological collections such as Liverpool, Glasgow, Edinburgh and Bristol. In all of these cities there is a university college of veterinary studies very close to a fairly large new complex, and there is a lot of exchange of ideas and information between the veterinary surgeons in the zoos and those in the universities. It is through these sorts of channels that the opportunities for veterinary surgeons arise.

There are some opportunities for research, but this depends on the institution. In somewhere like London, funded partially now, and later perhaps substantially, by government grant, there are quite wide opportunities for research — but for a limited number of people only. Including the director, there are only about five veterinary surgeons at London's Whipsnade Park and Regent's Park zoos, with two of these researching into such subjects as bacteriology and pathology, and at the same time assisting the zoo staff. Some zoos are run by zoological societies as charitable trusts to help the funding situation and these include Bristol, Chester, Edinburgh and London. Blackpool and some of the Irish zoos are owned by the local authority and the work simply involves looking after the animals. However, in most zoos there are some facilities for minor clinical research, depending on the wealth of the zoo authority.

If a local authority does decide to build and run a zoo, it may simply take on a local veterinary surgeon in practice. Salaries are low compared with general practice, and although it is an extremely interesting job, the veterinary surgeon would normally need to do other work to supplement his or her income to bring it up to a reasonable professional living. In some cases there is no permanent veterinary surgeon for a small zoo, and the local practice is called in as and when necessary, or the work may be contracted out to a private practice. In a university town, the bacteriology and pathology department of the university may be consulted for diagnostic work and the large animal operating facilities at the veterinary faculty used if there is a surgical requirement for something that is extremely complicated or large and difficult. A veterinary surgeon at the university may be appointed as consultant to the zoo.

The BVA zoological group has meetings twice a year to discuss the treatment of zoo animals which are open to any veterinary surgeon with an interest in zoos, and gradually a pool of information has been built up. Over the last ten years many more books on zoo medicine have been produced and there is a lot more reference material available. To help veterinary students, staff of zoos connected to universities do some teaching.

Zoos Abroad

Although zoo jobs in the UK are limited, in some areas of the world it is a different picture, particularly in the developing countries where zoos are now becoming part of their educational and social programmes. In the Middle East and Far East particularly, the new zoo development is seen almost as a status symbol. In the Far East, Malaysia, Singapore and the Pacific Basin they are now starting to have an interest in zoological species and, as a result of this, they are tending to look for zoological expertise in the areas where it is most long-standing — that is, in Western Europe and America.

Some jobs abroad are very well paid; in Saudi Arabia, for instance, and the USA, too, although they normally prefer to take on American graduates. Most Middle Eastern and Far Eastern posts are well paid. However, one has to take into account the fact that such a job does demand some degree of sacrifice. You would be living in a country that has a totally different culture and way of life, and would normally be under instruction from a national of the country and so would not really be your own boss.

Contracts normally run for three years — which could mean abrupt unemployment. For many people it is an ideal way of life, which they enjoy, with perhaps house boys, big houses, servants and big cars; returning to the UK after that type of life means accepting a lower standard of living. Although it is a contractual post, if the contract is regularly renewed it can become permanent and very satisfying for someone who fits in well, although opportunities are limited.

Entering Zoo Work

The best way to get into zoo medicine would be to show an interest in zoo work during the stay at college, and to try to get some experience working in a zoo during the veterinary college course, or to work with a zoo veterinary surgeon. This would help in making useful contacts. Then, towards the end of the college course, before graduating, look for an opportunity for a job in one of the zoos in the UK where you can gain experience. With two years' experience you can then apply for jobs abroad — it is unlikely that a new graduate direct from college would be able to walk straight into a job with a zoo overseas. Veterinary surgeons who have already worked overseas with one of the development agencies and may have gained further qualifications, perhaps from one of the universities overseas, may be successful in finding a zoo curator's post in one of the developing countries.

The Royal Army Veterinary Corps (RAVC)

Although the Army no longer uses large numbers of horses, or mules, as it did in the past, it does now rely on dogs to do a great deal of important work. At any one time there are 200 dogs at the Army Dog Training School who will eventually be used to protect military camps and installations, search for terrorist weapons and explosives, detect mines, track fugitives and assist the Military Police. Horses are still on the Army payroll, of course, for use on ceremonial occasions by regiments such as the Household Cavalry and the King's Troop, Royal Horse Artillery. Regimental mascots, such as goats, provide variety — and, for some reason, pig farms. Army veterinary surgeons working abroad may also have charge of the saddle horses, and the servicemen's own pets.

The RAVC veterinary officers (VOs) have a wide range of responsibilities within their field. They choose the dogs and horses, and are in charge of training them as well as their management and veterinary care. There is an emphasis on preventive medicine, including regular examinations of the animals, and the facilities for medical and surgical treatment are of a high standard, with well-equipped surgeries and hospitals and trained assistants. The surgeries have their own facilities for clinical and pathological investigation and diagnostic tests, and there is a back-up service provided by the Army Veterinary Laboratory at Aldershot which carries out more specialised procedures and research.

The VOs are in charge of their own budgets for such items as drugs, dressings and expendable items. As Army officers, the VOs are in command of other people, who will include dog trainers, farriers, veterinary assistants, clerks, riding instructors, kennelmaids and grooms.

There is naturally plenty of opportunity for postings abroad, and there is a great deal of dog-work in Northern Ireland. In Hong Kong over 200 dogs are used, and there the commanding officer also has the responsibility of advising on border security and rabies prevention. There are also permanent units in Germany and Cyprus. Other countries visited regularly or occasionally include Holland, West Germany, Gibraltar, Nepal, Thailand, Oman, Australia and the Falklands. In countries with regular units overseas, VOs must have a knowledge of the local import and export regulations; and in certain units they undertake the inspection of meat for human consumption. With so much work overseas, the Army veterinary surgeon is very often involved in the area of tropical disease.

Opportunities for research exist at Aldershot and other establishments, into subjects such as service dog nutrition, veterinary public health and biological warfare defence.

The RAVC accepts new graduates straight from veterinary school; they must be passed by an Army medical board. On appointment, an officer is granted a short service commission, of which normally four years are on the active list and four years are on the reserve. During the period on the active list, male officers can apply to be granted a regular commission and, if accepted, can then expect a career until the age of 58; special regular commissions are also available for selected female officers. The rank of captain is accorded to all VOs on commissioning. Veterinary surgeons with postgraduate experience have this taken into account up to a maximum of four years' seniority for pay. A two- to three-year posting system ensures that each officer gains experience in a number of different appointments.

The newly commissioned VO reports first to the RAVC training centre where he or she prepares for the first appointment, receiving training in dog handling, methods of instruction, OVS (red meat; radiological protection) and sometimes basic equitation; he or she will also attend a four-week military orientation course at Sandhurst.

Army pay is computed on a daily rate — highly applicable to veterinary officers, whose work with animals means that they will be working a seven-day week (with compensating days off duty). Pay is for 365 days a year. Rates for a captain are £28.56 per day (1984 rates) going up to £29.33 after one year. Further details are available from the Ministry of Defence, Army Veterinary and Remount Services (address on page 108).

Chapter 5

The Animal Welfare Societies

Those animal welfare societies that do employ veterinary surgeons on a full-time basis cannot, of course, afford to pay very high salaries. Often local practitioners give advice and treatment on a consultancy basis.

PDSA

The People's Dispensary for Sick Animals has around 157 veterinary surgeons on its staff — far more than any other welfare organisation. They work in the 57 animal treatment centres that are owned by the PDSA and sited in virtually every major industrial town and city of the country, from Aberdeen to Plymouth.

The Society was founded in 1917 and is a registered charity established to provide free veterinary treatment for sick and injured animals whose owners are unable to afford private veterinary fees. Nowadays old age pensioners living on small fixed incomes are the most frequent users of the service, but it also gives help to other low-income pet owners, including the unemployed, and to children. Education in the proper care for pet animals is one of the PDSA's major aims.

The Society's treatment centres are equipped with modern X-ray units and other diagnostic aids, comprehensive surgical and laboratory equipment, preparation rooms, operating theatres, post-operative recovery rooms and aftercare wards. All provide a 24-hour emergency service, but all animals must be taken to the centre — there are no house calls. Treatment is free to those owners who cannot afford private fees, but they can make a voluntary contribution when they take their pets for treatment. The work is nearly all with small animals. The starting salary for veterinary officers is between £6,000 and £7,000, plus car and allowances. Regional veterinary officers receive up to about £18,000 plus car and allowances.

There is a PDSA auxiliary service in some communities where there is no treatment centre; it is provided by local veterinary practices acting on the PDSA's behalf. The service is available only to those in receipt of one or more state benefits living within certain clearly defined boundaries.

The PDSA also does some work abroad: in Morocco, Egypt and South Africa.

RSPCA

The Royal Society for the Prevention of Cruelty to Animals has several animal homes, clinics, sanctuaries and hospitals of its own, with the work undertaken there provided by local veterinary practices. The very few veterinary surgeons employed by the Society full time are based either at their major hospitals, or at their headquarters to provide a back-up service for the workers in the field, and to provide them with veterinary advice.

Blue Cross

The Blue Cross has three fully equipped animal hospitals, two in London and one in Grimsby, which are staffed by full-time veterinary staff, including veterinary surgeons. Outlying clinics are supervised by visiting veterinary surgeons who liaise with local private practitioners.

Chapter 6
Opportunities Overseas

The register of the members of the Royal College of Veterinary Surgeons, which is published each year, shows that a sizeable proportion of the members are working abroad. Although many of these are not graduates of British colleges, having graduated abroad and then taken the Royal College's examination for membership, there are also many veterinary surgeons from Britain who have gone overseas, and in fact there is plenty of work abroad.

Very often veterinary surgeons go abroad in their own right and set up in private practice in the same way that they would in the UK. Or they may join organisations such as the Hong Kong Jockey Club, or the International Livestock Centre for Africa, in Kenya. Industry also has veterinary surgeons abroad; major companies will often have a veterinary presence in overseas countries.

Another important and challenging area of work, totally different from the type of work in the UK, is in the developing countries, where veterinary surgeons combine with other experts to help develop food resources. This can involve field or laboratory work. The Overseas Development Administration (ODA) is a large government organisation that sends people overseas in this capacity, and VSO is well known as a group that arranges for young people to go to developing countries on a voluntary basis, at local rates of pay.

Work in the developing countries is normally of a non-permanent nature, although the ODA does have one type of contract for up to ten years. A drawback of working overseas can be that veterinary surgeons may become out of touch with developments at home, although this would not be a problem for people working in general practice.

The Overseas Committee of the BVA now offers travel grants of around £250 to four students each year, to help towards travel costs. The scheme has been going for only a short time, but already they have had students going to Nepal, Peru and Harare where they have had the opportunity to work in various institutes, veterinary schools and large practices. They get the flavour of the country as students, and the BVA committee hopes they will be stimulated to return in the future.

General Practice

Since December 1980, veterinary surgeons from the UK have been free to put up their plate in any member state of the EEC, and vets from the other member states have been able to come to work in the UK; in fact there are a few who are already in practice here. However, language and other problems have so far proved to be difficult hurdles for British veterinary surgeons wanting to practise in Europe, and there are very few working there at the moment.

There are no extra examinations necessary for any veterinary surgeons who want to move from one state to another within the EEC, but those from further afield who want to come to the UK may have to take the Royal College's Diploma of Membership before being allowed to practise here — unless they have graduated from certain specified universities in Australia, Canada, South Africa and New Zealand, in which case they can practise without further examination. British vets who want to practise in the USA or Canada must take local state examinations before they can be registered, to satisfy the state's examining board that they are of reasonable standing academically to practise. The examinations would have to be taken and passed by the vet before leaving the UK — but they do not normally present any difficulty. A complication is that taking and passing the examination that allows you to practise in one state does not apply in the other states of the USA or Canada — being registered in Ontario does not also give the right to practise in Alberta, and if necessary another examination would have to be taken.

There are British veterinary surgeons working in many of what were once the colonies, where there is less likely to be a language barrier. Normally people in private practice go abroad because they have an ambition to travel overseas, and there is no special financial incentive — but there is financial security, in that practice work is as well paid as similar work in the UK, certainly in the USA and Canada, and usually, too, in Australia (which is described as being oversubscribed with veterinary surgeons at the moment) and New Zealand.

British Volunteer Agencies

About ten qualified veterinary surgeons are sent overseas each year by Voluntary Service Overseas (VSO). The postings are always for two years and they will take only qualified vets, preferring people who have some experience, preferably of large animal practice, either during their degree course or afterwards. Normally the vets are young, and understand that although they will get very interesting work and experience while they are abroad, they can become slightly out of touch with what is happening in the UK. They would have more responsibility than they would at home at the same age, and it is a very good first step for those wanting to do overseas work, for instance with the ODA.

It is not necessarily a good step for those who want to come back to the UK, because although they would certainly find a job, it would not be at the same stage of their career as they would have reached had they stayed in the UK, so it would be wrong to assume that service with a volunteer development agency helps your career. It does help, however, in terms of personal qualities; and in terms of professional qualities it would develop some skills, but leave other skills undeveloped.

Normally the work is of a very practical type, mainly with large animals, and principally on disease prevention, rather than curative work. The animals dealt with are cattle, sheep and goats, and poultry. There is not normally any survey work — finding out what diseases are present, and collecting and analysing the data.

The veterinary graduate is often part of a general agricultural project, doing not just straight veterinary work, but putting his or her skills and knowledge at the disposal of the whole development scheme.

To give illustrations of what volunteer vets find themselves doing, here are brief descriptions of two requests that were made for volunteers with veterinary degrees during 1984: one came from Bangladesh, and the veterinary surgeon was needed to set up a village veterinary centre with training and extension services; to supervise part-time animal husbandry workers; to promote the proper techniques of artificial insemination, chicken rearing, goats, cows and draught animals; to set up a Newcastle disease vaccination programme for poultry; to set up a hybrid breeding programme with cockerels and a foot and mouth vaccination programme. The volunteer needed a degree or diploma in veterinary science plus experience — and the ability to ride a motorbike was essential!

Another request came from Fiji, from a farm management co-operative association that needed a veterinary officer to train farm managers and villagers on about ten farms in nutrition, hygiene, breeding and disease prevention, and to assist the farm managers in setting up feeding and breeding programmes. Common problems were quoted as: scours, internal worms, ringworm, calving, mastitis, pregnancy diagnosis and tuberculosis. It was hoped that the volunteer would train the farm managers to a sufficient level of skill within two years so that no replacement would be needed. There was the chance of a great deal of flexibility, initiative and self-reliance in this job — but it also called for the ability to travel throughout the country, putting up with remote and basic conditions.

do so. In the Muslim countries of the Middle East, where a lot of ODA work is, it is very difficult for women to get jobs. Although of the five annual PTAS studentships, two have been women in each year recently, ODA do suggest that women should do a laboratory course because it is easier to place women in laboratories than in field jobs — but they often prefer to do field work. In the Yemen Arab Republic, for instance, where there is a large ODA project, it would not be possible for women to work, except in the laboratory. But although a veterinary surgeon may have done the laboratory course, the veterinary degree qualifies a man or woman to do field work if a job comes up in a country where there are no restrictions, such as any of the Southern Africa or Latin American countries. A laboratory course, therefore, widens the possibilities rather than narrowing them.

When recruiting, the ODA is not looking for excessive idealism, described as contra-indicated, although people who go abroad do so because they feel they want to help. Tenacity is a looked-for quality, because there can be a great deal of frustration and disillusion caused by lack of sufficient funds and also of appreciation. (A vet in Vanuatu in the Pacific islands recently sent an urgent request to the BVA overseas committee for tuberculin testing syringes, because she had a project to do there and nothing to do it with.) A sense of humour is also needed, an equable temperament, and adaptability.

Food and Agriculture Organisation (FAO)

The FAO is based in Rome and is an agency of the United Nations particularly concerned with food and agriculture, improving the condition of rural populations and raising the levels of nutrition in developing countries.

There is a sizeable number of British vets working with FAO, who may be sent overseas as specialists for anything from three to four days or three to four years. They are recruited through the ODA, by the Administration's International Recruitment Unit (IRU), which is at their East Kilbride department (address on page 108).

Returned Volunteer Action (RVA)

RVA is an independent organisation of and for British volunteers and ex-volunteers. Their leaflet *Thinking about Volunteering?* (25p in stamps, plus sae) contains hints to help would-be volunteers make an informed decision on going overseas as a volunteer, and there is a programme of activities to support returned volunteers (address on page 108).

Universities

Information about postgraduate study at Commonwealth universities and academic posts is available from the Association of Commonwealth Universities.

Students wishing to do postgraduate research abroad are advised to consult the High Commission or Embassy of the country in which they are interested, as well as their head of department at university and the *Commonwealth Universities Yearbook* in their university's reference library.

Academic posts may be advertised in papers such as the *Times Higher Educational Supplement*, the *Guardian* or *The Veterinary Record* by the ACU's appointments service.

The British Council, which is mainly concerned with promoting Britain overseas, also recruits teachers for posts in universities and training colleges abroad.

Case Studies

Michael worked overseas for about 13 years with the ODA.

> I was in Botswana, El Salvador and Ethiopia, and all were very different. I was a field veterinary officer in Botswana and a veterinary investigation officer in both Ethiopia and El Salvador, finding out what diseases occur, what are the most important ones, and how to control them. In Ethiopia I worked mainly in liver fluke and trypanosomiasis (sleeping sickness) which occurs where there are tsetse flies.
>
> Ethiopia had everything from sunstroke to frostbite and we dealt with rinderpest, foot and mouth disease and other diseases which don't occur in England. It was a fascinating five years and I did feel I'd achieved something, although it would be in the longer term. I was there during the Somali/

Ethiopian war and through the first famine, which was a horrifying but fascinating experience. When people throw themselves into your Land Rover and ask for water — nothing else — it's horrifying; but by treating sheep twice a year for liver fluke we could reduce sheep mortality by half and double people's cash income. A difficulty was getting the treatment to them, off the main roads. On trypanosomiasis we managed to keep cattle alive to plough land in areas where people said we couldn't, so they were able to grow crops and we settled several thousand from famine areas — and they were able to make a cash income as well. The differences — the culture, the poverty — are all stressful, and one can find it very difficult, but I was fascinated by the culture of Ethiopia.

In Botswana I was controlling foot and mouth disease in cattle and in many ways it was a simple project in that Botswana's main source of foreign exchange was the export of meat to Europe, and that export was based entirely on the control of foot and mouth disease. If they got the disease, they lost the export market.

I was in El Salvador for two years and the war was very near, which didn't help. I enjoyed learning the language [Spanish] and about the different culture. I was looking at tick-borne diseases and the control of them in cattle. During that time I did a veterinary science course at Edinburgh for a year. My wife enjoyed it thoroughly and prefers being overseas in many ways. She is an infant teacher and in each of the countries taught at kindergarten (she ran her own in Botswana) or at the English School.

John did a tour with the VSO.

I was working for a Sri Lankan development organisation called Christian Workers' Fellowship that had set up several projects dotted over the island in areas where research was needed. I was working at a rural service centre where the fellowship had bought and was running a farm to gain an insight into the problems affecting the rural sector. They became involved in dairying and became the base of a milk co-operative. They decided to apply for a vet through VSO because one of the limiting factors in dairy development in that area was the poor availability of veterinary service, with the result that the farmers had not invested in their dairy enterprises.

By the time I got there the dairy industry had collapsed because of the increased cost of concentrate feed and a low fixed price for the milk, so I was too late. I found myself dealing with just a small number of animal and survey type work on milk production, fertility and husbandry, which had not been done intensively in that kind of area, and we helped in the surveys being undertaken by the local veterinary school and veterinary institute, which were nearby. The farmers were not used to treating animals, so if an animal needed three days' treatment I had to go back every day and see it, whereas in this country you would treat on the first day and then prescribe treatment for the farmer to give it and never see it again, so it was satisfying to follow cases right through. On the other hand there were very few animals so that I was not gaining as much clinical experience as one would need at that stage in one's career. It's very important to consolidate what you've learnt, so from that point of view it was not so good. However, I enjoyed my time in Sri Lanka and don't regret doing it.

It took me quite a long time to get a job back in the UK. The veterinary profession seems to be rather reactionary about anybody who has done anything different; I had to apply to a lot of practices and found I couldn't even compete with recent graduates. I was unemployed for six months altogether. However, I am now in a mixed practice, working mainly with cattle, so it has worked out very well. I hope to go abroad again to work in development with the ODA, who finance the tropical veterinary medicine course at Edinburgh University.

Part 2

Chapter 7

Training to be a Veterinary Surgeon

Places of Study

There are six veterinary schools in the UK where you can study for a veterinary degree, and one in Dublin. All are attached to universities. Those in England are: Bristol, Cambridge, Liverpool and London, and the two in Scotland are at Edinburgh and Glasgow. All the courses last for five years except for the one at Cambridge, which is a longer, six-year course. Not all the veterinary schools follow exactly the same syllabus and even the titles of the courses and the name of the final degree are different. At Cambridge, University College, Dublin, London and Edinburgh the name of the course is 'veterinary medicine'. At the other three schools it is called 'veterinary science'.

At Bristol you would be awarded the degree of Bachelor of Veterinary Science (BVSc); at Cambridge you are awarded a Bachelor of Arts degree (BA) in science after the first part of the course, and then continue with the second part for the further degree of Bachelor of Veterinary Medicine (VetMB), ending up as a BA, VetMB; at Dublin it is a degree in Veterinary Medicine (MVB); at Edinburgh the degree is Bachelor of Veterinary Medicine and Surgery (BVM&S) and an honours degree of Bachelor of Science in Veterinary Science (BSc(VetSc)); Glasgow has the degree of Bachelor of Veterinary Medicine and Surgery (BVMS), with Honours or Commendation if special merit has been shown throughout the course; Liverpool's is a Bachelor of Veterinary Science (BVSc) and at the Royal Veterinary College, London, the degree is Bachelor of

Veterinary Medicine (BVetMed). As most are different, you can tell at a glance where someone has studied.

There are courses of further study in veterinary science. At Liverpool, for example, further degrees and diplomas are: Master of Veterinary Science (MVSc), Doctor of Veterinary Science (DVSc), Master of Animal Science (MAnimSc), Diploma in Bovine Reproduction (DBR) and Diploma in Equine Reproduction (DER). Postgraduates at the colleges can also study for a PhD. There are alternatively separate degree courses that can be taken by postgraduates who are interested in a particular scientific aspect of veterinary work, and who want to specialise or gain further qualifications.

Once students have graduated from university as veterinary surgeons they are not allowed to practise until they have become members of the Royal College of Veterinary Surgeons, which they can apply to become at the end of the course. This gives them further letters after their name: MRCVS, which are all-important to the veterinary surgeon who wants to practise.

The number of places for veterinary students at university are limited, so that the numbers qualifying keep the profession at a steady level (in the last 140 years the number of veterinary surgeons registered has increased to only 11,000). This does mean that new graduates can be sure of finding some sort of job, although recent government cutbacks and the decline in national prosperity have reduced vacancies in some sectors. It does also mean, however, that it is very difficult to get one of the small number (390) of places available. In 1984, in the UK (excluding Dublin), there were 330 places and 322 graduates qualified, so the drop-out rate is low. Competition for these places is very stiff indeed, a ratio of around 16 : 1, and only those with very good grades stand a chance of finding a place, and even those with acceptable grades may find there is simply no room. Unfortunately, although there are other jobs that involve work with animals, none is in any way close to the standard of a veterinary surgeon's, and cannot compare in salary. Those who cannot get into veterinary school are often advised to try for another university course in a similar discipline, if they are good at science, so at the time of applying it is advisable to list three veterinary schools on the UCCA form, and use the other two choices on the form to apply for such subjects as natural sciences, medical biology, microbiology and immunology, biochemistry, physiology, agriculture, animal production or a similar related subject.

Personal Qualities

Apart from the ability to achieve a high standard of work academically, people who want to become veterinary surgeons need a scientific and observant mind, and must be able to keep up their study throughout the course. Those who want to work with animals in practice of some kind eventually must have an understanding of animals and a real interest in caring for them, and be able to handle them in a calm and confident way, even when their patients are difficult and distressed. As owners are of importance, too, a broadminded ability to communicate with the public, especially with awkward or difficult members, is a necessary asset. In private practice it is no good being an excellent academic vet if you are such a cold personality that people do not like to come and see you. General mixed practice work (ie farm and pet animals) means being able to be on duty, sometimes, for 24 hours a day and at weekends as well as weekdays, and the veterinary surgeon has to be physically active, too, if a great deal of the work is out of doors. Those who will eventually go into research need to be strongly motivated towards it, and be blessed with the ability to come up again and again with worthwhile projects to work on.

Experience with Animals

The veterinary schools at the universities expect those applying for the veterinary courses to have had experience with animals; ideally they are looking for people with a lot of motivation, who perhaps have grown up on a farm, had their own horses, and looked after them themselves. Obviously this cannot apply to many students, but it is advisable for them to work with animals and to spend time with a veterinary surgeon in practice before applying for a university place. The universities will want to see this kind of information on the application form, and the RVC, London, insists on two weeks spent with a veterinarian before entry to the college, either in private practice or in some other branch of the profession.

Working with a veterinary surgeon in this way gives a much better understanding of the pressures, long hours and hard work involved than reading the Herriot books does — they were set in a period when a vet's life was quite different from the way it is today. It also tests whether the prospective student has a genuine vocation and concern for the welfare of animals that are sick, rather than a sentimental love of them when they are healthy. Unfortunately, even people who are strongly motivated and academically well-qualified may find that they simply cannot work with animals because of some allergy or sensitivity.

Experience with animals can be obtained by working in kennels, stables, farms, helping in a local practice, etc, and the sooner it is started during the years at school, the better. Once a student has the provisional offer of a place at a veterinary school, a veterinary surgeon will normally be prepared to let him or her spend time working in the practice.

Requirements for University Admission

There are no hard and fast rules about grades, but normally you must have a minimum of three passes at A level, with AAB grades in subjects such as biology, chemistry, mathematics, physics and zoology usually at the first attempt. Candidates for Bristol and RVC, London, can offer subjects outside this range. At Edinburgh and RVC, London, physical science is an alternative to chemistry. Physics is an alternative to a mathematics subject at Bristol, Edinburgh,

Glasgow and RVC, London; if mathematics is offered, a good O level pass in physics is necessary. Bristol, Edinburgh and RVC, London, require biology or zoology; Glasgow requires biology, and Liverpool requires either biology, zoology or mathematics. Cambridge requires chemistry plus any two of physics, mathematics and biology (zoology/botany). Candidates for Cambridge can offer physical science instead of chemistry and physics. Universities may insist on first-time passes.

Edinburgh and Glasgow require those with SCE qualifications to have five Higher grades at AAABB including chemistry at A and physics and biology at A or B. Candidates unable to offer physics may offer mathematics instead, but they must have a good O level physics pass.

Where a subject is not offered at A level, O level passes may be necessary: English or an approved test in English are required at Cambridge, Dublin, Liverpool, Edinburgh and Glasgow. At Cambridge, Dublin and Edinburgh an approved language in addition to English is necessary. Physics is required at Bristol and Liverpool; mathematics or science at Cambridge. Edinburgh requires a good O grade in mathematics and English, with another language; Glasgow accepts a good O grade in physics instead of a Higher grade, provided the candidate has Higher grade mathematics.

These subjects are in addition to the university's own entrance requirements, which will include a lower age limit as well as academic qualifications. Requirements may be altered, so it is as well to write to the university for full details.

Scottish candidates with SCE qualifications cannot enter the veterinary courses at Liverpool and London, as both universities accept only GCE passes, but students with Certificate of Sixth Year Studies examination passes may be accepted at Liverpool.

How to Apply

Applications to universities are made through the Universities Central Council on Admissions (UCCA), but there

are different provisions for the universities of Glasgow and
Edinburgh. Information is given in the UCCA handbook
How to Apply for Admission to a University, which is
essential for all applicants; a copy of this will be kept by
schools. Applicants for Cambridge need to make a direct
approach to the departmental secretary of the department
of veterinary medicine to find out about the college
entrance procedure; Cambridge also has an earlier closing
date for applications than the other universities. At Cambridge the date is 30 September, and at the other universities, 15 December; but early application is advisable in
all cases.

University College, Dublin, mainly accepts only students
from the Republic of Ireland, although there is a limited
number of places available for applicants from Northern
Ireland and from countries in the Irish bi-lateral aid programme.

As universities are less likely to accept applicants who
place them in fourth or fifth place in order of preference on
the UCCA application, the wise course for veterinary
students would be to list universities in alphabetical order,
indicating three preferences at the head of their list for
veterinary degree courses, and perhaps using the other two
spaces to indicate alternative courses that they would like
to take within the university if they are unsuccessful in
getting into veterinary school.

Before entering Cambridge University, it is possible to
do an interim year after leaving school, as long as plenty of
notice is given. The same thing can apply at Bristol and
Edinburgh. The booklet, 'A Year Off', published by CRAC,
gives ideas and information on voluntary service, work
camps and summer projects, paid work and study courses in
Britain and abroad (£1.95).

The College Courses

Veterinary students spend the first part of their five- or
six-year course learning about the make-up of healthy
animals in depth, and this is known as the pre-clinical

part of the course. Animal management, dealing in all aspects of the recognition, housing and handling of the common breeds of domestic animals, is also taught at varying times from the first to the fourth year of the course. The para-clinical subjects, including pathology, bacteriology, virology, parasitology and nutrition come before the final clinical subjects of medicine and surgery. The colleges follow differing schedules, but all will cover anatomy — the structure of different species of animals and birds; physiology — normal functioning of the animal's body; biochemistry — natural chemical processes in plant and animal life; pathology — diseases (their causes, effects and outcome); medicine — diagnosis of disease, remedial substances and dietetics; pharmacology — action and effects of drugs on the body; surgery — operative procedures, radiography, anaesthesia; bacteriology — disease-producing organisms in decomposing matter; parasitology — parasites such as worms, lice, fleas, ticks, etc, that infest the body, externally or internally; animal husbandry — farm management, grassland and pasturage, housing of livestock; practice management — general administration of a veterinary practice; and legal and public health aspects.

At many universities there is a chance to break off for a year during the course so as to study one particular discipline, or subject, in depth for a BSc in a subject such as anatomy, biochemistry, cell biology, genetics, physiology or pharmacology. At Cambridge the increased emphasis on pre-clinical sciences in the first part of the course leads to the separate BA science degree, and is the reason why students with a particular interest in the sciences would apply for Cambridge with its longer course.

At Cambridge and Dublin, veterinary students study during the pre-clinical years with medical students, and at Bristol the same is true in the subject of biochemistry; other subjects are taught separately, although within the medical school. At London and Edinburgh, the longest-established veterinary schools, and Glasgow and Liverpool, study is almost entirely separated from that of other students within the universities.

Students work with live animals during the latter, clinical part of the course. The colleges have veterinary hospitals where small animals are seen that normally come for treatment from the area near the college, and large animals are seen at the 'field station'. Veterinary schools have their own farms (or farms owned by the universities) and also have access to other farms as part of an agricultural practice that belongs to the school, or through an arrangement with local veterinary surgeons. There are also institutions connected with the different schools that influence the education of the students. For instance, Edinburgh has an important centre of tropical medicine and offers postgraduate MSc and diploma courses in tropical veterinary medicine as well as in neurophysiology and in state veterinary medicine, and students benefit from being taught by staff experienced in these fields. There are also three AFRC research institutes and a Veterinary Investigation Centre (VIC).

Bristol has its own practice teaching unit and is close to an AFRC research institute and to a laboratory researching into trypanosomiasis, a group of tropical parasitic diseases, and which, like Edinburgh's Centre for Tropical Veterinary Medicine, is well known to veterinary surgeons connected with work overseas.

Cambridge has a VI centre adjoining, and also close links with two AFRC research institutes and with the Animal Health Trust centres at Newmarket.

Liverpool also has a VIC associated with it, and parasitology teaching is linked with the Liverpool School of Tropical Medicine; its field station is in an important dairying area. RVC, London, of course, is near the zoo as well as several medical and research units; the field station is in Hertfordshire — and the girls may be sent to a farm in Wales where their smaller hands are useful in helping with a flock of special sheep that has problems in lambing. (The intake of women to veterinary colleges is normally the same as that of men — 50 : 50.)

All veterinary schools insist on up to 12 weeks of approved experience in livestock husbandry, and six months' practical veterinary experience during the course. This has to be taken during the vacations. The type of experience varies but can include work in abattoirs, as well as on farms, in stables and kennels and time with a practising veterinary surgeon.

More detailed information, including details of grants, is available from the universities themselves. Also the RCVS's booklet, 'A Career as a Veterinary Surgeon', and the CRAC Degree Course Guide, 'Veterinary Science'.

Case Study

Mike:

> I had no future mapped out and stumbled into veterinary medicine, although I'd succeeded in getting places at medical and dental schools. I didn't really fancy being a doctor and quite liked animals; two of my good friends were going to be vets and someone had told me it was a good life — on reflection it sounds terribly naive, but then most of us are at seventeen! College was very enjoyable for me scholastically and socially. The vet course is hard, though, and no one gets by without working hard. There were 70 students in our first year but by the final year we were down to 45. The course prepared one well for general practice as a jack-of-all-trades, but would not do for some of the increasingly specialised cattle, equine and small animal practices around now. The veterinary school I was at seemed also to be lacking in sufficient practical material and I was not initially very good at some crucial basic techniques, so took my first job in a practice where I would get the chance to improve them.
>
> Of the five years spent in training, 30 weeks each year were spent at the university and for the first two years one must find work on sheep, cattle and pig farms for 25 weeks of the 44 weeks' holiday. This time off, seeing practice and working on farms, could be either a waste of time or an excellent experience depending on the farmer or vet one was with. In some cases we were slave labour for the farmers. Only my lambing time experience taught me anything of veterinary use — the other farm periods only taught me how lucky I was not to be a farm worker, and what farmers think of vets! Only one practice gave me valuable help, and that was because there were young assistants there who remembered what it was like to be green, and so helped me a lot.
>
> In all we sat some 130 examinations of which we had to pass 17. I enjoyed the courses, with the exception of statistics, which I really detested!

Chapter 8

The Professional Associations

The Royal College of Veterinary Surgeons (RCVS)

The RCVS had its beginnings in the first two veterinary schools founded in this country. The first was opened in London as early as 1791 and had as its principal a French veterinary surgeon, trained at the veterinary school of Lyons. The second veterinary school was founded by William Dick in Edinburgh in 1823. The history of animal medicine was older, of course — animals had been invaluable as transport, as well as food, from the earliest times — and there was a trade guild, formed some time before 1356, of the Master Marshals of London (marshals were originally in charge of a noble household's horses).

The graduates of the two veterinary schools were worried about the activities of untrained quack animal surgeons, and petitioned Queen Victoria for a Royal Charter incorporating them as the Royal College of Veterinary Surgeons. The petition was granted with a Royal Charter in 1844, restricting the title 'veterinary surgeon' to members of the College only.

Originally all veterinary students were examined by the College itself, but since 1948 the universities have been responsible for examining the students and awarding the veterinary degree: it is holding the degree that confers upon the holder the right to membership of the RCVS, and to registration in the Register of Veterinary Surgeons maintained by the College — and thereby the right to practise veterinary surgery in the UK. No one who is not registered with the College may practise in the UK, even though he or she may have a veterinary degree.

The Royal College is the governing body of the veterinary profession in the United Kingdom. It has statutory powers and responsibilities regarding veterinary education and the maintenance of ethical standards within the profession, as well as responsibility for keeping the Register of Veterinary Surgeons. It receives the statutory powers both from the first Royal Charter and from later ones, and from several Acts of Parliament.

On admission to membership of the College, the new graduate becomes entitled to vote in elections for the Council of the College, which is responsible for aspects of veterinary education and for ethics and discipline — it is possible for a veterinary surgeon to be struck off the Register, for a limited period or permanently.

A fee has to be paid to the College when the new graduate is admitted to the Register, and there are fees paid annually afterwards. Veterinary surgeons from other EEC countries are free to register with the RCVS without further examination and therefore to practise in the UK, and veterinary surgeons from the UK can practise in member countries of the EEC, which of course includes the Republic of Ireland. The College still examines for a number of postgraduate qualifications including the Fellowship of the RCVS, the diploma in veterinary anaesthesia and the diploma in veterinary radiology. With the increasing amount of specialisation within the profession, there are other diplomas planned for the future in other veterinary disciplines and in relation to particular species.

The College has a comprehensive library: the Royal College of Veterinary Surgeons' Wellcome Library, at the College's headquarters in Belgrave Square, London. It has an historical collection of veterinary literature, and a modern working reference library for the use of College members. Details of scholarships and other awards made by the College are given in the RCVS booklet 'A Career as a Veterinary Surgeon'.

The British Veterinary Association (BVA)

After the Royal Charter was granted that allowed the

formation of the RCVS, local associations of veterinary surgeons were formed, some of the oldest being those of the West of Scotland, the Lancashire, the Yorkshire and the Midlands counties, until by 1880 there were 15 associations plus three abroad. The first National Veterinary Congress was held in London, with the help of the 18 associations, in 1881, and a British National Veterinary Association was set up, which held meetings every year. In 1952 the association became the British Veterinary Association, and now has 28 'territorial' divisions on the lines of the first 18, and 19 special interest groups. There are 8,000 members.

The territorial groups of the BVA cover every region, from the Cornwall Veterinary Association to the North of Scotland Division. The special interest groups include the Association of Veterinary Students and the Society of Women Veterinary Surgeons, as well as associations for members specialising in cattle, horses, poultry, pigs, sheep, goats, pet animals, public health, and so forth.

The BVA exists to promote the interests of its members and monitors the activities of government, local authorities, other professional organisations, animal welfare societies, and so on, and to keep abreast of new developments.

The BVA also publishes three major journals. *The Veterinary Record*, which was bought in 1920, is the only weekly veterinary journal in the world. It keeps the members informed about the latest scientific achievements as well as other news of interest to the veterinary surgeon. It publishes papers and articles, book reviews and letters from members. Pages at the back have advertisements for assistants, partnerships, practices to sell, locum appointments and jobs in universities, pharmaceutical companies and development agencies in the UK and abroad.

In Practice is published bi-monthly and is designed to keep the practitioner up to date in clinical matters; *Research in Veterinary Science*, also bi-monthly, is a journal in which members and others record the results of their research. The BVA also publishes the *Equine Veterinary Journal* on behalf of the BVA division, the British Equine Veterinary Association.

Chapter 9
Useful Addresses

British Veterinary Association, 7 Mansfield Street,
    London W1M 0AT
Royal College of Veterinary Surgeons (RCVS), 32 Belgrave Square,
    London SW1X 8QP

State Veterinary Services

Civil Service Commission, Alencon Link, Basingstoke RG21 1JB
Civil Service Commission, Rosepark House, Upper Newtownards
    Road, Belfast BT4 3NR, Northern Ireland
Civil Service Commission, Lower Grand Canal Street, Dublin 2,
    Ireland
Department of Agriculture, Dundonald House, Upper
    Newtownards Road, Belfast BT4 3SB, Northern Ireland
Department of Agriculture, Agriculture House, Dublin 2, Ireland
Department of Agriculture for Scotland, St Andrew's House,
    Regent Road, Edinburgh EH1 3DA
Meat and Livestock Commission, PO Box 44, Queensway House,
    Bletchley, Milton Keynes MK2 2EF
Ministry of Agriculture, Fisheries and Food, Great Westminster
    House, Horseferry Road, London SW1P 2AE
Regional Veterinary Officer (Staff) MAFF, Block B, Hook Rise
    South, Tolworth, Surbiton, Surrey KT6 7NF (for
    information about veterinary officer posts)
The Director, Central Veterinary Laboratory, New Haw,
    Weybridge, Surrey (for information about research officer posts)

Teaching and Research

Agricultural and Food Research Council, 160 Great Portland Street,
    London W1N 6DT
Agricultural Institute, 19 Sandymount Avenue, Dublin 4, Ireland
Animal Health Trust, Headquarters, Lanwades Hall, Kennett,
    Nr Newmarket, Suffolk CB8 7PN
Institute of Biology, 41 Queen's Gate, London SW7 5HU

Horserace Betting Levy Board, 17-23 Southampton Row,
    London WC1B 5HH
Leverhulme Trust, Research Awards Advisory Committee,
    15-19 New Fetter Lane, London EC4A 1NR
Medical Research Council, 20 Park Crescent, London W1N 4AL
Natural Environment Research Council, Polaris House, North Star
    Avenue, Swindon, Wiltshire
Science Research Council, Central Office, PO Box 18,
    Swindon SN1 5BW
Wellcome Trust, 1 Park Square West, London NW1 4LJ

RAVC

Royal Army Veterinary Corps, Ministry of Defence, Army
    Veterinary and Remount Services, Government Buildings,
    Droitwich, Worcestershire WR9 8AU

Welfare Societies

The Blue Cross, Animals Hospital, Hugh Street,
    London SW1V 1QQ
People's Dispensary for Sick Animals, PDSA House, South Street,
    Dorking, Surrey RH4 2LB
The Royal Society for the Prevention of Cruelty to Animals,
    The Causeway, Horsham, West Sussex

Overseas Work

British Volunteer Programme, 22 Coleman Fields, London N1 7AG
International Voluntary Service, Ceresole House, 53 Regent Road,
    Leicester LE1 6YL
Overseas Development Administration, International Recruitment
    Unit, Abercrombie House, Eaglesham Road, East Kilbride,
    Glasgow G75 8EA
Returned Volunteer Action, 1 Amwell Street, London EC1R 1UL
United Nations Association International Service, 3 Whitehall
    Court, London SW1A 2EL
Voluntary Service Overseas, 9 Belgrave Square, London SW1X 8PW

Training
Universities and Veterinary Schools

The Registrar, University of Bristol, Senate House,
    Bristol BS8 1TH
The Cambridge Intercollegiate Applications Office, Kellet Lodge,
    Tennis Court Road, Cambridge CB2 1QJ
The Administrative Secretary, Department of Clinical Veterinary
    Medicine, University of Cambridge, Madingley Road,
    Cambridge CB3 0ES

The Dean, Faculty of Veterinary Medicine, Royal (Dick) School of
Veterinary Studies, University of Edinburgh, Summerhall,
Edinburgh EH9 1QJ

The Chairman of the Admissions Committee, Faculty of Veterinary
Medicine, University of Glasgow, Veterinary School, Bearsden
Road, Bearsden, Glasgow G61 1QH

The Sub-Dean, Faculty of Veterinary Science, University of
Liverpool, PO Box 147, Liverpool L69 3BX

The Registrar, Royal Veterinary College, University of London,
Royal College Street, London NW1 0TU

The Dean, Faculty of Veterinary Medicine, University College
Dublin, National University of Ireland, Veterinary College of
Ireland, Ballsbridge, Dublin 4

Other Relevant Bodies

Association of Commonwealth Universities, 36 Gordon Square,
London WC1H 0PF

Careers Research and Advisory Centre (CRAC), Hobsons Press,
Bateman Street, Cambridge CB2 1LZ

Department of Education and Science, Elizabeth House, York
Road, London SE1 7PH

Scottish Education Department, 2 South Charlotte Street,
Edinburgh EH2 4AW

Universities Central Council on Admissions (UCCA), PO Box 28,
Cheltenham GL50 1HY

US-UK Educational Commission, 6 Porter Street,
London W1M 2HR

Chapter 10

Further Reading

General Texts

A Career as a Veterinary Surgeon, from the Royal College of
  Veterinary Surgeons, 32 Belgrave Square, London SW1X 8QP;
  £2.00.

Animal Care and Veterinary Science, No 111 in Choice of Careers
  Series by Careers and Occupational Information Centre (COIC)
  from HMSO, Government Bookshop, 49 High Holborn,
  London WC1V 6HB. Available in Career Centres.

A Year Off, a guide to opportunities for work, travel and voluntary
  service, from Careers Research and Advisory Centre (CRAC),
  Hobsons Press, Bateman Street, Cambridge CB2 1LZ; £1.95.

Careers for Veterinary Graduates in the State Veterinary Service,
  from the Establishment Officer, Ministry of Agriculture,
  Fisheries and Food, Great Westminster House, Horseferry
  Road, London SW1P 2AE.

Care of Animals, from the COIC Working In series, COIC, Sales
  Department, Freepost, Sheffield S1 4BR; 99p plus 25p p & p.
  CB3 8RG; 95p plus 25p p & p

Guide to partnerships in veterinary practice, from the British
  Veterinary Association, 7 Mansfield Street, London W1M 0AT;
  £1.00.

How to Apply for Admission to a University, published by
  Universities Central Council on Admissions (UCCA), PO Box 28,
  Cheltenham GL50 1HY. Copies are normally available at
  schools.

Model agreements between principals and assistants, from the
  BVA (address above); £1.00.

Running Your Own Boarding Kennels, S. Zabawa, published by
  Kogan Page, 120 Pentonville Road, London N1 9JN.

Veterinary Science Degree Course Guide, from CRAC (address
  above); £2.85.

Undergraduate Grant Guides

Grants to Students. A Brief Guide, from the Department of
  Education and Science, Elizabeth House, York Road,
  London SE1 7PH.

Guide to Students' Allowances, from the Scottish Department of
  Education, 2 South Charlotte Street, Edinburgh EH2 4AW.

*Memorandum — Grants to Enable Students to Follow Courses of
  Higher Education*, from the Irish Department of Education,
  Rathgael House, Balco Road, Bangor, County Down BT19 2PR.